CONFESSIONS OF A
COMMUNITY NURSE

Lucy Spencer

<u>Dedication</u>

For S, for keeping me motivated and reminding me of my capabilities, for picking me up when I worked beyond exhaustion, for listening to the tears as well as the smiles, and for being my inner strength.

xxx

Disclaimer

Lucy Spencer is a pseudonym for a Registered Adult Nurse working in the East Midlands.

This book is intended as a memoir of sorts, to attempt to give a glimpse into my own personal experiences as I transitioned from student nurse through to newly qualified nurse in a community setting. The humour is sometimes tongue-in-cheek and there is no intention to put down the National Health Service in any way. It is not intended to suggest medical advice – if you have any health concerns, please contact the appropriate healthcare service.

Effort has been made to preserve confidentiality and anonymity wherever possible.

Contents

<u>Introduction</u>

No organisation can escape the politics, budgeting issues, resourcing difficulties and hiccups in providing the ultimate service, and the health service is no exception. But what is it that makes these industries still operative and appealing for people to work for?

It's because of the people involved that are still, despite the daily challenges they face, passionate about the work they do and committed to making it successful. Those people who say "I'm not in for the money" and genuinely mean it. And let's face it, the majority of those who work for the National Health Service are certainly not in it for the money.

This book is an honest account of my experiences as a student nurse to a newly qualified professional working in the community. It is not intended to whistleblow or denigrate the NHS in any way – I have been supported fantastically from start to present by tutors, mentors, colleagues and most other people I've come into contact with over the years.

I've learned something from everyone I've worked alongside, from support workers to porters to patients (and I've personally been all three). Whether it's maintaining a good work-life balance, controlling the trolleys on the way from A&E to X-ray so I don't inadvertently cause more injury by smashing my patient into a doorframe, or even just making the perfect cup of tea for Mrs A at number 68 (my

1

greatest achievement yet), I've learned valuable lessons that someday I can pass on to my own students and colleagues.

The NHS is under massive pressures, from waiting lists to bed management, recruitment and retention concerns to service cuts. But aside from this, one thing I remain sure of is that I am proud to work for the NHS. Even in the toughest of times, the NHS family pull together remarkably to put the patients' needs first. Administrative staff, nurses, porters, paramedics, doctors, clinical educators, housekeepers; everyone contributes invaluably to keep the cogs of the NHS well-oiled despite the troubles we face, whether they are clinical or behind the scenes.

We are available 24 hours a day, 7 days a week to transport, nurse, resuscitate and counsel. We go out of our way to help you and if we can't, we will signpost you to someone who can. We provide life-saving treatment, manage debilitating symptoms and support patients and families struggling with illness. We assist in the arrival of new lives into the world, and hold the hands of patients at the end. From birth to death, we are there for every stage of life in between, for minutes or months, or sometimes years. We clean up a cut forehead, reassure a worried mother and provide years of therapy to help someone walk again. We will laugh with you, we will cry with you, and we will sit in silence with you, if that's what you need. We see our work family more than our own, we suffer verbal and physical abuse, and we put on weight because chocolate and cake is still the best way to say thank you. We care, we console, and we do it all without judgement. We will encourage you to drink plenty of fluids and get excited when you pass urine, even though our own bladders haven't been emptied for nine hours. We will stress the importance of sleep and rest for recovery, but lay awake ourselves wondering how you're getting on hours after our shifts have finished.

I am a nurse. I have looked into the eyes of a baby minutes after birth, and I have cared for people after life-sustaining surgery. I have rejoiced with a patient who has just had his first independent shower in three years, and I have recognised sepsis and saved lives. I have smiled when patients are discharged because they are better, and I have brushed the teeth of those too ill to do it themselves. On the other side of the coin, I have performed last offices both in expected and unexpected deaths. I have provided a silent cup of tea to a mother coming to terms with the fact her son will never wake up. I have recognised a medication error made by a junior doctor who hasn't slept for 28 hours when I myself, haven't slept for 21. I have been kicked in the stomach, scratched, bitten and sworn at. I have also been hugged, thanked, complimented and 'requested'. I have many an affectionate nickname from patients and colleagues, and I've met my best friends through healthcare. I have been an anxious patient and a concerned relative. I have been a learner and a teacher. I am proud of my profession and I am proud of the NHS as a whole.

To everybody, sincerely, thank you.

I'm Not Ready

The third year of my nursing degree all but killed me off. I was overwhelmed with the number of assignments all due in at the same time, disheartened with how my grades had dipped a bit (not so much the smart arse I was in the first and second years!) and confused by the fact I had gained so much knowledge and experience and yet, I felt the least ready to be a registered health professional than ever.

In Year Two, I made a decision that is single-handedly responsible for my love of energy drinks (yes I know); I started working night shifts as clinical support at a local hospital. I hoped to increase my experience (and bank balance) and get a better understanding of the areas I hadn't experienced on placement. The majority of my training placements were 'community-based' and I felt that, if I was to work my first job on a ward, I would be like a rabbit caught in the headlights, right before it got smushed into a shadow.

So, alongside my nursing degree, I worked in orthopaedics (bones), maternity (babies), intensive care (really poorly people) and oncology (cancer), before finally finding my comfort zone in the Coronary Care Unit (intensive care for the heart) and later, Accident and Emergency. These two work areas were the making of me as a student about to transition into registration.

In CCU (Coronary Care Unit) I was the only clinical support on shift and became proficient in fluid balance (what goes in and what comes out), resuscitation protocols, recognition of the deteriorating patient and ECG recording. All skills I hadn't yet had chance to practice during training except inside the classroom. These skills I took with me to A&E, where I further developed my communication and interpersonal skills as well as clinical competencies.

Working nights around my studies meant I usually worked Friday and Saturday nights at the main hospital in the county, and it's quite safe to say if nothing else (fatigue-induced giggles and big black circles around my eyes notwithstanding), it dramatically improved my personal confidence as well as my trust in my abilities as a healthcare professional. So to all those nursing students out there looking for part-time work (which is probably most of you now the powers-that-be have ditched the bursary), going on the bank at a local healthcare Trust is much more beneficial to you as a person as well as your career than working behind the bar in a student pub, serving five shots for the price of one. Chances are, if you work Friday nights in A&E, you'll see the same people anyway.

Three months into my third year of training, I was offered a position at that hospital in MEAU (Medical Emergency Assessment Unit). I was also lined up for Neonatal Intensive Care (poorly new-born babies). It was getting real now, the future was coming thick and fast. In a matter of months, I would no longer be the support – I would be the one needing it. Cue confidence and career crisis.

I've always been incredibly enthusiastic about emergency care and I loved working in A&E, even if I did crack my head on those bloody oxygen dials fifteen times an hour. I'd also worked with the ambulance service on voluntary shifts and this had served to reawaken my interest in Paramedic Science. In all honesty, I didn't even want to specifically be a nurse to begin with. At sixteen years old, it was only one of my career considerations, along with Forensic Medicine and Biomedical Science (both of which were more 'paperwork than people', and neither of which I felt passionate enough about to make a career of it). I looked into joining the Royal Air Force as a medic, but didn't fancy being a soldier first and foremost. It was only due to personal circumstances that I didn't apply to train as a paramedic when I was eighteen years old.

Ten years later, I found myself being a few months from completing my nursing training and still not having the faintest idea where to start building my career. I'd gained so much knowledge through study and experience at the hospital, but I wasn't 100% sure I wanted to work on a ward. Some days, I even wanted to abandon it all for a flight to Thailand to begin a semi-hedonistic lifestyle, backpacking around the tropics and letting the wind blow me where it will. These people who live in treehouses and survive on rice and coconuts make it look so easy…

I remember being told in my first year of study by a nurse, "Get your first job in A&E, ICU or MEAU, and you can work anywhere". That statement had stuck with me and although I understand the reasoning behind it, I'm one of those people who thoroughly enjoy one-to-one patient contact, something you don't necessarily get in the fast-paced environments. I was guaranteed my job in MEAU but applied for a position as a Community Nurse, a job I thought was much more 'me'. I applied, interviewed, accepted that job and the rest as they say, is history. End of book.

Just kidding.

Identity

Community Nurse, District Nurse, Practice Nurse on the road, Private Paramedic, Doctor Helper, Glorified Carer...

All terms I have heard used to describe the job I do. My official job title is 'Community Staff Nurse'. I work within a team of other community nurses (RNs/Trained) and healthcare assistants (HCAs/Untrained) under the lead of a District Nurse (DN). I've also just recently finished my preceptorship, meaning I've left the phase of increased support where I was also known as an NQN (Newly Qualified Nurse). As you can see, us medical lot love the abbreviations, particularly the unofficial ones we make up ourselves...

Bizarrely, all through my three years of training, I insisted I would never work as a community nurse due to the politics and pressures of the area (an opinion influenced by my training placements). I believe at one point, maybe after a particularly tough day, my words were "F**k that". That was mainly before my experiences in the hospital. Political issues and job pressures are everywhere, regardless of what speciality you work in. Looking back at my 'student views' of various areas to work in, one might wonder why I even became a nurse?! But from the bottom of my heart, I absolutely love it.

What's changed? Everything I love about nursing I am allowed to practise in such an autonomous role.

Being a registered nurse is quite different from being a student, even as a third year where you're expected to have minimal supervision only. Was it a case of wanting to run before I could walk? Possibly. Or was it the inability to see the difference I could make whilst training under tired nurses who had been jaded by the profession, who felt undervalued and overworked? Maybe.

After three years of working in very different specialities, I was able to reflect on the experiences I'd had, focus on my strengths and what I could bring to the table, analyse what it actually is that I love about nursing, and consider how I could develop my career skills, whilst at the same time, maybe attempt a life. Part of me perhaps felt 'stifled' as a student; I certainly felt more confident in a clinical support capacity. I could be doing something as clinical support and feel 100% competent but doing the exact same thing in a student nurse uniform, a big chunk of that confidence vanished. Being observed and assessed at every corner maybe gave me a little bit of performance anxiety.

As I matured through my training, I started to see nursing from an entirely different perspective. I now see things from angles I didn't even know were there. That's nursing in a nutshell: a lifelong learning opportunity. I fully support the decision to require a minimum of two years care experience before applying for nursing. I had years of care experience when I applied but a few I knew didn't and dropped out of the course because training wasn't what they expected. Not all of them were 'too posh to wash' but there were unfortunately some with that attitude. The number of students who dropped out during the first year of training was almost shocking – every time the register went round in lectures we could see the numbers dwindling from the previous week's session. I've heard a surprising amount of student nurses say they don't give personal care, that's not what they went into nursing to do. In my opinion, if that's what your patient needs, you do it.

Nursing in the community is working with people in their own surroundings. People don't live in hospitals – everything about their being changes. I want to nurse the person not their condition, and if that means providing personal care, then that is what I will do.

So anyway, in a quick overview before I digress too much, that's how I came to be a community nurse after graduation over any other type of nurse. I fought my way to the end of nursing school, doubting my own knowledge and skills far too many times to count, found my new comfort zone, stepped out of it, and discovered the reason why nurses come to work every day. Even though we are community nurses (and various other, often incorrect, associations of the word), we continue to work as a multidisciplinary team (MDT) to provide the best care for the patient. We work closely with GPs, social workers, occupational therapists, physiotherapists, mental health nurses, paramedics, the list go on…

What follows now is a collection of stories, written as a kind of blog with lots of internal monologue, in an attempt to open the door and give a sneak peek into life as a student nurse developing into a newly qualified community nurse. Some stories may seem like a rant (and have provided the perfect opportunity for reflection for revalidation!), but others may hopefully offer some insight into how rewarding this career path is. It is upsetting, it is exciting, and it is stressful – the daily combination of these things is part of the reason healthcare professionals develop a dark and sometimes morbid sense of humour as a coping mechanism (seeing as drinking on the job and swearing out loud at infuriating patients/relatives is a big no-no). As they say, if we didn't laugh, we'd cry. And I've done both. Sometimes on the same day.

Certain situations are repeated on the road more often than we'd like, and some recounts are an amalgamation of several very similar occurrences. Issues are universal across the field and in no way connected to any particular organisation or service provider; all views are my own and details have been changed to protect anonymity. Some of the humour is tongue-in-cheek and not intended to cause offence (although I know it will somewhere, I never could please everyone).

No Cardiac History?

During my first training placement, I was placed in a rural district nursing team and to be brutally honest, was absolutely terrified. I had none of the professional confidence I have now, I was practically scared of my own shadow. I had left the safety of the lecture theatres and was now a 'real' student nurse. After a few teething issues, mostly around my confidence, I started to settle in and looking back, it's shockingly clear how much I've developed and in certain ways, completely changed.

One day towards the end of the nine-week placement, my (absolutely fabulous) co-mentor and I visited a gentleman for a first visit. He had recently been discharged from hospital and brought home with him a little wound on his rear, caused by pressure damage. At first visits, we need to do full assessments; we have key questions to ask and depending on the answer, we may need to delve a bit more into it, a bit freestyle. Some call it 'professional curiosity' but basically it's just being really bloody nosy. This sugar-coated interrogation covers pretty much the life story of the patient, including medical history. We work through the body systems top to toe, any respiratory illness, any heart problems, any stomach issues etc. Now, we already know the answers to these because we have access to your records on the computer system. Asking you enables us to understand how much you understand, and how any conditions affect you personally.

We were talking through this assessment with the patient in an informal way, "any heart problems?" we asked. "Nope, fit as a fiddle me". Well, we know that's not quite true don't we, because we're seeing you in the first place, but he was insistent. He was still insistent when we found bottle upon bottle of cardiac medication in his kitchen cupboards. Pills for high blood pressure, angina spray, cholesterol tablets, you name it he was on it. If he didn't understand the nature of his health problems, it may take some work to get him to understand the nature of his pressure injury and wound healing.

Sometimes it pays to have a little bit of a nosy around the environment that we're in. Not just to be nosy of course, but if we're concerned about whether someone is eating properly, we'll have a quick scan of the cupboards and we always take note of what's in the fridge when we get your insulin pen/make you a cup of tea. We'll notice if your bed is so covered in clutter you can't possibly be sleeping in it. We make mental notes of fire hazards and environmental health risks. We can gain so much information about you without even asking, it's quite a skill. Nurses are inherently excellent readers of people; we possess high levels of intuition and, as my patients have found out, I **know** if you're lying to me, even if I don't know the truth just yet.

Some people get quite defensive when you suggest their living conditions aren't optimal to a healthy life, but if they have the capacity to make that decision, sometimes we have to just walk away and leave them to it. I visited a house once as a community RN and it was literally like a derelict shed. I didn't know if I should knock on the door before I stepped over it, and there were so many cobwebs I'm sure they alone would have been classed as a fire hazard. Piles of newspapers were everywhere you turned, and I half expected mice to be scurrying about or to find a litter of kittens tucked away somewhere (don't ask, I don't know why I genuinely thought this might be a possibility). There were fruit flies in the kitchen, hovering around old cabbage heads and grocery boxes, and I don't think any of the doors had handles. How anybody could live there is beyond me. I'm capable of getting cold in the middle of August, it must have been dreadful in the winter. But, he lived there and he was happy there. He had capacity to make that decision and surprisingly, the only reason we were there was to change a urinary catheter every twelve weeks. It takes some skill to adhere to the aseptic non-touch technique in that environment let me tell you!

Rose Cottage

When I started training and began caring for patients at the end of life, and even now, there's always the though at the back of your mind, what if today is **the** day? Quite miserable I know, but when people are quite close to the end, from the professional side, it's a little bit of a worry that you're going to be there when they go, or that you're going to walk in one day and they've already gone. Especially in the community when you can get quite 'attached' to people, it's that moment where you need to be professional and keep it together for the families, even though you may well be falling apart inside because you're the only professional there, with no back-up from other nurses and doctors that mill about on a ward.

At the start of my nursing career I'd seen precisely one dead (human) body, a resident in a care home I was working at when I was nineteen, and I was there as he took his last breath. I didn't really stay around much afterwards because I was needed on the floor while the senior staff took care of him, cleansing and shrouding. Aftercare of the deceased was definitely something I would have to experience (without sounding as though I was **waiting** for it) so I knew how I would react. Human emotions can be very unpredictable in new situations, particularly with ones we're uncomfortable with, and until you're in that situation for the first time, you'll never truly know how you'll react.

I decided to break through that wall in a controlled environment and got in touch with the mortuary manager at my local hospital. I arranged to spend the day with them during a post-mortem examination. I wasn't nervous as such, I was…something. I can't describe it. Curious? Intrigued? If anyone knows a less morbid way of saying excited, please let me know.

So it was on a sunny August morning that I marched down the darkest corridor in the world that, funnily enough, isn't signposted from the main hall, to the department known amongst hospital personnel as 'Rose Cottage', or 'The Cottage'. It's a bit more discreet on a ward filled with patients and relatives to request a porter to the cottage than it is to ask for a porter to the morgue. I had a pre-brief and kitted up: full length gown, shoe covers, gloves, the lot (well, except a face mask, which I asked for halfway through in an attempt to trick my mind into not smelling raw flesh). I'm not sure what I expected but it didn't match at all.

For a start, there were two bodies already on the slabs. I only ordered one. Apparently, this is done for time - pathologists don't routinely sit around waiting for people to go upstairs, they have meetings and work across other sites spanning a very large area. I was going to be working with the mortuary technician to start with – these are the people who do all of the 'dissection' work. To be suddenly faced with two bodies on two slabs, in a room that didn't resemble an operating theatre at all (this is one thing

I did think it would be like, not an old-fashioned sluice room) shut me up immediately. Was I ready for this? With a keen interest in forensic medicine for years, I realised if anything was going to put those anatomy textbooks into context, it was this. Yes, I was ready. I think.

With a speed that quite honestly astounded me, the bodies were opened up and 'emptied' ready for the pathologist to do his bit. The technician worked so quickly but so precisely, he was nearly finished before I had even grasped the concept that these were no longer living people. As a nurse, even when patients are unconscious, we still speak to them as though they can hear every word (well you just don't know really do you – after a motorbike accident, a relative can tell me almost everything about his stay in ICU, even hearing the conversation to turn off the ventilator). I had a million and one questions but it didn't feel right to ask in front of the 'patient'.

I won't go into too much detail about the post-mortems, I don't want to create any nightmares or existential crises, but once the pathologist arrived, with our backs to the empty shells that lay behind me, it was easier to view this part of the autopsy as a science lesson. I'd dissected lungs and hearts and eyeballs at school, and without a body attached, it was much easier to close myself off to where I actually was. The pathologist was excellent in his teaching, talking me through every step; why he cut certain organs in certain ways, what he was looking for, what he might find in certain diseases, clinical findings, asking me about the anatomy.

Despite having lungs and kidneys and a liver in front of me, I was most fascinated to see the ovaries in real life, and was surprised at how small they were. The only time I became a little overwhelmed was when we sliced the brain. That organ was what had made that person. All of their knowledge, their memories, everything that made their personality and kept their body alive all these years. The human body is an amazing system, life made possible by the brain which we were now slicing up like a piece of meat in a butchers.

By the time we had finished and established two causes of death, the first body was already 'put back together' and ready for the funeral home. Truly artists in their work, the incision sites were neat and would be easily hidden by hair and clothing, in case the family wished to view their loved one. Overall, an experience incredibly worthwhile in terms of anatomy study and processing my own thoughts on death, even though it stayed with me for at least two weeks afterwards, replaying in my head. I think it took my own brain a while to catch up and catalogue what I'd seen.

If I could witness autopsies without passing out or throwing up, I would have no problem performing hygiene care when patients passed on during my shift. As a nurse, I would never need the level of detachment those guys had – I guess they needed it to be able to sleep at night. I wonder how many people think about the mortuary team when they consider a patient's journey? It's a side of health and medicine I imagine people choose to be ignorant to. As a student, aside from making biology lectures 'come to life' so to speak, it encouraged a lot of reflection on my views of human mortality. It's not for everyone; I've known student nurses who hate the sight of blood let alone anything else, and I've seen the lovely grey colour their faces go after I tell them I've assisted with post-mortems.

On my way out of Rose Cottage, I noticed the freezer doors had ages on. Some were in weeks. I'm pleased I didn't attend on the day they did those ones.

Life After Death

As a nurse (and blood donor) you'd probably expect that I'd be an organ donor as well. In actual fact, at the start of writing this book, I wasn't. At the end of writing this book, my name is on the Organ Donation Register. Partially anyway. I won't donate my eyes.

I'd be quite happy to accept an organ if I needed it so it's only fair that I give something I no longer need after death. But in all honesty, it wasn't a clear-cut decision to make. After a lot of internal conversation about the why's and why not's, I have so far agreed to donate certain organs but not others at the present time. I wonder if it's because I consider myself a reasonably spiritual person, in terms of 'other side' spiritual. It's an aspect of my personality that conflicts with having two Bachelor of **Science** degrees. Nobody has ever proven the existence or non-existence of life after death – the Egyptians were massive fans of it as demonstrated in their after-death rituals, belief in Gods of the Underworld and putting organs in Canopic jars. Many superstitions and practices around the world are influenced by the possibility of life after death, from coins on the eyelids by the ancient Greeks to pay the ferryman, to removing mirrors to avoid trapping the soul on its journey to the afterlife. As a woman of science maybe I should say, once we're dead, we're dead. As a woman of spirituality maybe I should say we're all reincarnated and other such blah blah blah. In reality, I'm somewhere in between. Logically I know I won't need my organs but there was something inside that just felt hesitant about not going in one piece.

A relative has told me that they would donate everything except their heart, because they feel quite strongly that the heart makes the person, and being without a heart even in death unsettles them. It's interesting how different people have different views about these things when you start enquiring about it. I've opted to **not** donate my corneas for a reason I can't quite verbalise – perhaps the expression 'the eyes are the windows to the soul' resonates quite strongly with me. If I'm not having all of my body go with me wherever I might end up, I at least want to see where I'm going.

I suppose I was a bit concerned by the fact that everything must move quite quickly in order to have a viable organ to donate, and I worried about the impact on my family. For successful transplantation, organs must be kept 'alive' and what better way to keep organs alive than to keep them in the body they grew up in. This 'beating-heart donation' made me think about how my family would cope. I know they'd be proud that I would be continuing to save lives even after death, but my body would have to be kept warm, pink and with a pulse, albeit mechanically ventilated. Even if I was dead dead, I don't think my family would be able to accept that was the case in the midst of grief. I know I would have trouble processing it, even as someone who knows what needs to happen.

I cared for a 24-year-old once who had attempted suicide by hanging but had been 'interrupted'. Unfortunately, the interruption came too late but in a way, too soon. The patient had not completed suicide in that they hadn't been pronounced dead at the scene, but the event had starved their brain of oxygen for so long, it would never recover. It was so damaged, the body could only just sustain breathing and circulation – not quite 'braindead' but irreversibly and catastrophically hurt.

The patient came to us on the ward from intensive care, to pass away peacefully in a private side room. I will never forget how my heart bled for the mother, who sat by her child's bedside 24/7 just waiting for their body to get too tired and take its last breath. That was the only prognosis, there was absolutely no hope of improvement. All I could do was make Mum cups of tea and ensure she was warm enough as she sat crunched up in a chair next to the bed, not moving for days. Sadly, this was a case where organ donation wouldn't have helped, and the air was thick with grief in that side room, even though biologically, the patient was still alive. I can't imagine how difficult it must be to see a loved one's body showing signs of life when in fact, they are never going to wake up. I left that shift feeling quite deeply emotionally affected.

There was a study published in the very early 1900's by a doctor in America that found that one out of six bodies weighed exactly at the point of death, appeared to 'lose' just over 20 grams. Obviously one in six is hardly concrete evidence of a soul but it's certainly put the theory out there, and until someone proves otherwise, I am not agreeing with either side of the life after death debate.

Providing Instant Access

Over the past four years, I've worked with a lot of people with substance abuse problems, whether it's been in A&E, with the substance recovery team, or in the community. From alcohol to codeine to crack addicts, I've developed a very keen nose for cannabis and can smell when someone uses heroin. I've also seen the lengths to which drug users will go in their desperation for their next fix.

In Year One of my training, I was working on a medical ward and one of the four patients in my bay, was a young woman admitted with cellulitis following ulcerated legs. Her legs were ulcerated as a complication of her intravenous heroin addiction and injecting into any vein she could find. She was on a methadone programme which the ward nurses administered whilst she was an inpatient; most of the day she was asleep but became quite active when it was time for her next dose. Sadly, many addicts continue to take heroin whilst being on methadone programmes, even though they know they're not supposed to.

I was changing bed linen one shift and noticed her sat on the edge of her bed trying to put mascara on. It was my first encounter of someone with an active heroin addiction and it was a really bizarre thing to watch. It was almost as if she moved in such slow motion, the concentration of putting on her make-up had her quite literally falling asleep, wand in hand. I woke her up a couple of times and she carried on trying as though she hadn't just phased out to the world for a few seconds. I honestly believe if she were to look into a mirror, she would have started talking to her reflection and asked it who it was.

All in all, she was quite compliant with treatment and on the days where she was relatively lucid, she enjoyed telling me about her children, whom she no longer had access to. This changed quite dramatically on one particular day when her partner visited and the difference in her was unbelievable. She had gone from being in some sort of opiate-induced zombie state, to all of a sudden being desperate to get off the ward 'for a cigarette'. For a start, she was connected to oxygen so for us to let her disappear off to smoke a cigarette whilst sat on an oxygen tank would have been really irresponsible. The second issue we had was that she had a central line inserted (for reasons I can't remember now). Call us distrusting but something just didn't sit right with allowing a previously half-comatose patient who just so happened to be an IV drug user, to leave the ward now her boyfriend (who was probably her drug dealer as well) had showed up. There was instant access to her bloodstream through this line without the need to find a vein to inject into – it would essentially drop the hit right next to her heart.

We tried to distract her in every way possible whilst we sought further guidance from the doctor. Unfortunately, due to obligations around mental capacity and no deprivation of liberty safeguarding in place, there was nothing we could do to stop her leaving the ward, other than watch her go and hope they weren't going to go and stick a load of heroin into the port site. Or blow themselves up in a ball of oxygen cylinder.

The next year I came across this woman again whilst I was working with the drug and alcohol recovery team. She was attending the service for ongoing support, having come off heroin and finished methadone. She was clean of drugs and had put on so much weight I had to double-take. She was so different from the gaunt fragile figure I had seen ten months previously. She no longer spoke with a slur and I found out she was working and had regained access to her children. That story was a happy ending – it's so satisfying to see how services like that can make such a difference to someone's life. I can't understand how it can be justified to axe organisations in funding cuts when they can quite literally turn somebody's world around.

Year Two – Cardiac Speciality

Second year of nursing training and I had a placement at a specialist unit that has raised its county's survival rates of out-of-hospital cardiac arrests from 5% to nearly 50% - that's around 900%. Nationwide, the survival rate is 5-9.6%. That's an outstanding achievement; what an absolute pleasure to work with such an amazing team! With two specialist labs, routine and emergency cardiac procedures are carried out by the hospital's cardiac consultants, with emergencies sometimes by bypassing A&E all together, which is better for patient outcomes and department flow.

I spent most of my time in the recovery bays; I admitted people for planned angioplasties (a stent in the heart to reopen a blocked blood vessel – can be a day case procedure) as well as pacemaker insertions, and I cared for patients after their procedure through to their discharge either to the ward or back home. Monitoring vital signs and ensuring patients didn't bleed to death in front of me if their groin plug came out, the work was varied and certainly kept me on my toes.

During the stenting procedure, X-rays are used to guide a catheter into the radial artery in the wrist, up and into the heart to pop the stent in place (a bit like a wire tunnel that keeps the artery open). The vessel in the wrist is closed afterwards by a tight inflatable band that is slowly deflated over a period of time to allow the artery to 'seal' itself. Sometimes, either due to anatomy, difficulties in insertion or consultant preference, the catheter is inserted through the femoral artery in the groin. Here, the artery is a little too big to seal itself shut (and it only takes minutes to die from blood loss if it's ruptured), so a 'plug' is inserted which degrades itself. All very clever stuff until the patient laughs or sits up too quickly too soon, and the plug pops out. With no band in place here, the patient is at risk of fatal haemorrhage. Solution? Nurse stands with fist shoved in groin until bleeding stops. An event that kind of takes your breath away, quite literally being that pressure between life and death.

What I also found interesting is that, despite being in the middle of a heart attack, some patients were surprisingly upbeat. I remember being the scrub nurse's assistant in one emergency (heart attack brought in by the paramedics) and the patient spent the whole, quite literally life-saving procedure, singing. Anything to take their minds off it I suppose. Some patients didn't make it, but most did and were taken to ICU (Intensive Care Unit) or CCU, my soon-to-be stomping ground. While some patients threw up from a combination of pain and medication, some didn't even realise they were having a heart attack. These patients were mostly women and no, this isn't a dig at common sense, it's fact, although as a woman, I am tempted to say under my breath that it's because we are too busy in life to let a little thing like a heart attack get in the way. But of course, that's not medically or politically correct.

What I didn't miss about this placement, bar the thirteen hours on my feet, was the six tonnes of lead we had to wear in the labs. In the midst of a very hot summer, the lab was a popular choice amongst staff because of the ventilation and cooling systems required to keep the equipment working correctly (but far too cold for me). Because of the almost constant use of X-rays (the entire procedure is guided by radiographers using contrast solution), we had to wear lead aprons covering our bodies and a lead collar around our necks. It certainly gives you backache standing in that get-up for all day shifts. I still don't know how I carried all that weight around when I can't even support myself in a press-up posture and lift my own body weight. Thanks legs.

<u>Amazing Things</u>

One of my favourite things to do during my training, in between the six million words of assignments I had to write and the hours on placement/on shift, was spend time with the ambulance service. I wasn't paid and it was completely voluntary but it satisfied two purposes – being part of an emergency care team on the road (as I'd wanted all those years ago) and with the camaraderie between crewmates, it's just so much fun, and I learn the most when it's fun.

Working with my usual crew one evening, we were called to a care home where a resident had had an unwitnessed fall and bashed his head, resulting in quite an impressive bruise-bump to his forehead. We were under the lead of a fabulous paramedic that night who set about attempting to gain a history from the care home staff (who didn't know much, having not long started their shift, and clearly it wasn't explained during handover). The ECA (Emergency Care Assistant) and myself were sat chatting with a resident who was so confused he didn't know where he was, but he said that he loved music, particularly the piano. Somehow, we ended up walking him over to the piano which, almost conveniently, was on the other side of the room. "Did he play?" we wondered. May seem an odd wondering but I've had one single patient who has had careers as a doctor, an engineer, a detective…

Oh my, did he play! He played the most beautiful piece of music, not one note out of place (saying that, all of them could have been out of place, I wouldn't have known). The man had dementia so far on, he didn't know his own name, needed support to walk, and had fingers gnarled by the degeneration of arthritis, but in front of that piano, it all just disappeared. His hands moved with fluid-like grace across the keys, his eyes closed, and he was lost in the moment, in his memories. My colleague and I were blown away, we weren't expecting that at all, it literally rendered us speechless.

Once he had finished playing and accepted the huge round of applause from us, he returned to being that confused, frail old man we'd supported walking ten feet across the room, and we assisted him to sit back in the chair. He couldn't remember who he was or why he was in the care home, but he remembered that he used to be a music teacher and he remembered exactly how to play the piano when he was sat in front of it. It's amazing what the mind forgets and what it remembers with dementia. I guess it's just finding that link to connect.

Welcome to the Third Year

The first day of my third and final year of my nursing degree and it was almost as if I was selected for some kind of baptism by fire. Not a baby first year anymore, not a middle student who can just about get away with not being sure, I was a third year, soon to be qualified nurse, and the Universe decided I needed a shove into independence. If I was going to lose my 'responsible clinician' virginity, it was now. Not on placement or in the lecture theatres, but cycling home from University.

Full of fabulous thoughts in my post-summer holiday refreshed mind about how I was really going to get my head down this year, it's my last chance to start getting ready for the big wide world etc. I was in a world of my own biking down a cycle path through some fields on my way home. Up in front of me I saw someone sat on the side of the path. Didn't think anything of it, it's just someone having a rest, so I didn't slow down and carried on thinking about how I was going to get my arse into gear. Getting closer, I saw it was an elderly lady and a young woman. Getting even closer, there was blood. There was a lot of blood. I slammed my brakes on so hard I'm surprised I didn't go flying over the handlebars into the hedge myself. The elderly lady had come off her bike and literally snapped the bones of her forearm in two (or four depending on your anatomical knowledge). I threw my bike to the side of the path and introduced myself, making sure to mention I was a **student** nurse.

As far as cycling injuries go, it was reasonably impressive. The lady must have been in her 80's and had a 'Miss Daisy' bike with a basket so (I assumed tut tut) she couldn't have been going that fast, but she had fallen off, landed funny on her hand and broke her arm quite spectacularly. I saw the blood and then I saw the bones. Both of them were protruding out of her lower arm, just above her wrist. She was in and out of consciousness and waving the damaged arm about in between, spattering blood all over, but she was able to talk to me every now and then. Despite me asking though, she didn't keep her arm still (and given the pain she must have been in, I'm not entirely surprised). I tried to improvise. The woman had newspapers in her bike basket but that was it. No shoelaces or string or anything, so I had to simply rest her arm on the papers in the hopes it would avoid her getting any more floor muck in it and wiggling her hand right off her wrist. Legs raised, reassurance given, no further visible injuries but unable to rule out head injury (wear a helmet please people).

The young woman was on the phone to 999 but she couldn't describe exactly where we were to direct the paramedics to us. They were in a pub car park the other side of the river (now is not the time boys), the other side of the dual carriageway, and we were on the cycle route underneath the main road, hidden by trees and completely obscured. I took the woman's phone and ran as fast as my little legs could carry me, back up to the dual carriageway. I have never run so fast in my life and didn't actually think I was capable of running at such speed but here I was. I could see the paramedics in the car park but, due to four lanes of vehicles going at 70mph between us, they couldn't see me. I was stood waving my arms around like a lunatic, having every lorry driver beeping their horns at me as they went past – no I'm not waving at you. I gave up talking to the person on the phone, I would have to go and fetch the guys in green myself. More running.

I finally got to them, without needing their help myself, and led them to our casualty. People walking by slowed down but didn't stop, but there was enough of us now that they didn't need to. We had gained a first responder and these days, I'm surprised that the passers-by didn't pull out their mobile phones and take pictures.

The paramedics threw me some gloves and I set about taking blood pressure and pulse rate, keeping her arm as still as possible whilst they went about doing their other checks. At the minute, there didn't seem to be any compromise in the blood supply to her broken arm but there was no way they'd get an ambulance along the cycle path – there were bollards in place all along the route to avoid just that. "Stretcher?" they wondered. "Unlikely" I replied. The ambulance was still parked opposite and underneath the dual carriageway. The Air Ambulance was going to have to come.

By now, the woman was slightly more comfortable after pain relief but I was off on my travels again – running off along the path to lead the air team to where we were. They had landed the helicopter in the nearest accessible field which was a good half a mile away. When I set off cycling that morning, I did not count on getting as much cardio exercise in one day. I arrived back at the scene of the accident with the sky doctors in tow (at least I didn't have to carry all their kit on my back like they did – I would have ended up like an overturned tortoise). They decided, nope she's not going up in the air, so it was up to me again to go running back up to the main road and wave my arms around like a puppet once again, directing the ambulance to the closest point of entry to the cycle path. Even with the blues and sirens blaring, I could tell by the amount of time it took them to get to me that the traffic was not being kind. **Move out of the f**king way!!** They eventually parked on the hard shoulder and were bringing the stretcher down to the patient.

It took four of us to push the stretcher back up the hill once the patient was strapped in, and then we had to lift it up over the barriers. Off she went to hospital. The young woman went with her and, as I lived close by, I left my number and told her that I would take the lady's bike with me for safe-keeping. But not before cleaning up in the air ambulance because by this time, I was covered in blood from where the patient was waving her arm about and at one point, amidst all the bodies helping, I almost fell backwards (thanks to fatigue in my thighs like you wouldn't believe) into a nice puddle of congealed blood, leaving my lower arms looking quite a mess. I wasn't about to walk through my quiet village streets looking like that.

When I got home, I crashed. The shakes came and I felt utterly exhausted. I had to throw my bloodied jeans away and I stood in the shower for about half an hour. The patient had fractured her arm so badly, it took months of surgery and rehabilitation at a specialist hand hospital before she was fully recovered. She was nice enough to text me three months after the accident and ask to come and see me to say thank you, and she brought me the biggest bunch of flowers I'd ever received. I was just doing my job that day, putting my training into practice, but the thanks were gratefully received. Not how I expected to end a day of lectures at University. Welcome to the third year.

One Night Four Drunks

Accident and Emergency on a Friday night is just the same as any other night – busy but bearable. Until kicking out time that is. More times than we'd like, cubicles are taken up with drunks sleeping it off. The thing with drunk people in the street though, is that you can't always be 100% sure without a trip to the ED, whether they are just drunk or if there's something else accounting for their aggressive behaviour and slurred speech. Blood sugars being at either end of the scale can do this, as can head injuries. So ambulance crews bring them in to be on the safe side, where it's confirmed that they are inebriated, but by then we're stuck with them because they've drank so much they can't stand on their own two feet. I remember one evening there were a fair few such patients in majors, and one in the corridor.

Patient 1 (in the corridor waiting for a cubicle with the paramedics) was a teenage (read, underage) girl crying her eyes out to her friend, worried that she was going to die as a direct result of inappropriately high heels. How the paramedic kept a straight face I have no idea – we have perfected the art of hiding ourselves while we roll our eyes thinking "don't be so dramatic, you got pissed up and fell over" (or PUFO). The most she would have been diagnosed with is a hangover in the morning. Following the reassurance that she was not in fact, going to die, I heard the most girly conversation in history; a true declaration of love for the best friend who had come in with an adolescent party-goer. If Jack and Rose won an award for the 'you jump I jump, I'll never let go' thing in Titanic, this show of feminine solidarity would have come a close runner up. Nothing shows friendship like two drunk teenagers telling each other they love each other in voices so high only dogs can hear them.

Patient 2 woke up in a cubicle and began to wander off, taking the full drip of intravenous fluids with him. I didn't manage to catch him in time before he'd ripped the cannula out of the back of his hand and spattered blood all over the floor, leading to a full clean up on aisle 3.

Patient 3 I believe was homeless, but had still found enough money to drink himself halfway to oblivion (cause or effect, not yet known) and kept throwing himself to the floor. When I refused to get him up, because at 3am my attitude was leaning towards 'you got yourself down there for the seventeenth time, you can get yourself back up', I was called every name under the sun as he declared to the entire department that I 'didn't like him'. Aside from protecting my back, I didn't really want my uniform soaked in urine, vomit, or a combination of the two.

Patient 4 was an 89-year-old woman who was dolled up to the nines and incredibly drunk, awaiting a bed on a ward after being brought in following a fall. Three cubicles taken up (a quarter of the ED majors capacity) by people who had drunk too much alcohol. Hospitals would benefit from 'sleep it off' wards as, most of the time, that's all these people need; most are brought in PUFO and just need a quick check that they are actually just drunk and nothing else is going on. But yet again, lack of funding puts brick walls up for this and 'drunk tanks' in city centres, designed to reduce the pressure on the ambulance and A&E services (which I think is an excellent idea).

Diversion

Alcohol isn't the only substance that demands the attention of ambulance crews. Drug users may also need the services of emergency personnel, and presentation can mean that crews are diverted.

Ambulances are dispatched on a priority basis – even if they've been sent to one call and are on their way, they can always be diverted en-route if they're the nearest crew. This happened on a night shift; we had just dropped one casualty off at Accident and Emergency and had been called up before leaving the ambulance bay, to attend a fall in a care home to the south of the city. The ambulance had pulled out of the hospital, gone down the road a little bit, and just after the first set of traffic lights, we were redirected. Non-responsive male, suspected drug intoxication at the city police station. As we were the nearest crew, off we went. The elderly resident in the care home would have to wait.

At the station, the patient was well-known to the police and had a history of trying to have them on. However, a patient is a patient regardless, and complacency could have led to this one time meaning a serious illness was overlooked. We were led through numerous gates, each one locked behind us, to a cell with a man lying on the floor, two police officers stood outside keeping watch over him. As random a thought as it was, this was the first time I had seen the inside of a police station let alone a police cell. High security mental hospitals, check, mortuaries, check, but I've still to this day never been inside a regular police cell again (thankfully?). I was given the choice to enter the cell or stand outside it, and given my experience with drug abusers, I knew people who had taken this kind of drug, 'Mamba', could be unpredictable and sometimes aggressive. The cell was small; it would be a squeeze for three medium-build men without me in there as well. I'd stand outside thank you.

The paramedics did their stuff, checking blood pressure, pulse, blood sugar levels, whilst talking to the patient, who remained flat out on the floor. The police officers explained that sometimes 'prisoners' can do this in an attempt to either buy themselves more thinking time, or delay investigations so far that they're thrown out due to lack of evidence (they hope). The emergency crew started their little tricks to try and get a response, because although the guy played a pretty good game, we weren't 100% convinced that he was indeed out for the count. Water was flicked in his face (his eyelids flickered), his hands were lifted and dropped over his head (conveniently never falling onto his face but swinging down to a comfortable position), and he continued to feign being unconscious. "That's it then lads, we'll have to take him in".

Whether the man had intended it or not, he was getting his ride to the hospital. Better to have him completely checked out than to take a chance, particularly with his history of street drug use. Although he was still pretending to be unconscious, and there was a police escort in the ambulance with him while he was handcuffed to the trolley, I still felt better sitting up front. Was I scared? I'm not sure. Fear of the unknown? Maybe. I figured that while I still had a choice (which the A&E staff wouldn't have), I'd please myself and keep myself out of harm's way. If he was to become fully conscious hyped up on street junk and agitated/aggressive, police offer sat next to him or not, I didn't want to be sat in the clinical seat half a foot away from him.

At the hospital, the man refused to walk (but provided enough muscle tone and resistance to reassure the crew that he was in fact, pretending) out of the ambulance, so he was given a wheelchair. He would likely be sent to a private waiting area rather than take up a bed in a cubicle. He played silly buggers moving to the wheelchair, although he did miraculously 'wake up' after a very stern telling off from the police officer who was obviously tired of his games every single Thursday night. I felt like **I'd** been told off, the officer was that serious. Drug addiction is a controversial topic – yes, support services are thin on the ground and addiction is beyond some people's control but then again, some people do not want to be helped, they enjoy that lifestyle and are not interested in changing it.

This guy would probably spend a few hours in A&E as a change of scenery from the police cell but illness won't make the police forget what you were at the station for in the first place, you're just delaying whatever's coming next while you enjoy your drug high. He did play an excellent performance, to not laugh would have been hard enough for me, but I suppose he'd had plenty of practice and I was never much of an actress. I never did find out about the resident who had fallen, the one who had to wait longer on the floor while we attended a time-wasting thespian who liked to dabble with illegal drugs.

Think Before You Speak

As a final year nursing student, I undertook my management placement (the one where you're basically an unregistered nurse for £4 an hour and your mentors get to sit and drink tea all day) on a day surgery ward. Here, patients came in for same day surgical procedures and were usually discharged later that day. I observed surgeries, delivered and collected patients from theatres, managed the bays from start to finish and completed all of the paperwork at warp speed, ready for the surgeon and anaesthetist to come and ask all of the same questions at the beginning each clinic list.

Day surgery also accommodated patients who came in for intravenous infusions and blood transfusions. Here, I perfected my cannulation skills on actual real people instead of model arms which, by the way, are much harder than the real thing and the fake blood gets **everywhere**. My fellow student and I made such a mess in the chemotherapy suite whilst practising one afternoon that I think we spent more time trying to hide the evidence and scrub it out of the wooden table (don't worry, the suite wasn't in use that day).

The key factor in taking blood and cannulating is that you base your vein selection on feeling rather than seeing. I've never missed a vein yet and I genuinely believe it's because I don't look for them. I've even had patients comment on the fact that I sometimes look to my side rather than at their arm when I'm searching. Sure, you look first, but then it's all in the ends of your fingers. Your own sense of touch will tell you where to go and how deep. Literally close your eyes and feel your way. I was being observed by my mentor one day and was preparing to cannulate a regular patient for an immunosuppressant infusion. I had already chosen the vein I was going to go for, but my mentor wasn't looking, missed how I made my choice, and advised me to look at all the possibilities and comment on the appearance of the blood vessels. So I had a look at both arms, up and down between wrist and elbow, and said (out loud as in, people actually heard me), "you're just fine all over".

Now, this couldn't have been an elderly man with hearing difficulties could it. No. This of course had to be a young, muscular man with arms you could treat like a dartboard and still hit the target, with absolutely nothing wrong with his hearing. Ground swallow me up now. The other student found it completely hilarious and needless to say, I had great difficulty looking the patient in the eye for the rest of the shift. The remaining three weeks of placement were filled with innuendos in the staff room and I thought they'd never let me forget my embarrassment, until my mentor, who was from south-east Asia with not perfect English language, insisted that as a leaving present, she was going to buy me a Magic Bullet in order for me to start my day right. She meant a Nutri-Bullet, the smoothie-maker (I hope!) but the preceding three weeks had just done me in and I had to leave the room. Yes, I am immature.

Sharp Scratch

Something I was taught throughout my student years and was in the habit of saying without even thinking was, right before inserting needles, "sharp scratch". I have no idea why. There's no evidence base. By rights, you should have explained what you're going to do before you do it in the first place, in order to gain informed consent. I'm not sure why it's drummed into the heads of students because:

- It is **never** just a scratch if you hate needles. If you hate needles, it's the equivalent of an amputation without anaesthetic. It's never just a scratch anyway but I suppose saying "just a little prick" is lining you up for embarrassment on the previous story's level.
- In my experience, 'sharp scratches' actually cause patients to become more tense and anxious, because they're waiting for it.

I'm not overly bothered about needles myself, except those ridiculously massive ones they use when you donate blood. I can't watch them go in, they're like knitting needles, but as much as I scrunch my face up, it's still not as bad as I think it will be. When it's me inserting needles, I just do it, before the patient has too much time to think about it. By the time they've commented 'ouch' or some other such alien noise, it's done.

Bliss is ignorance springs to mind.

Blues and Bleurghs

Patients in the back of an ambulance have a double challenge to face – 1) they're (usually) ill enough to warrant being in the back of an ambulance anyway and 2) if anything is going to make you feel like throwing up your lunch, it's being in the back of an ambulance on a long trip cross-country. Whether it was because I was sat in the clinical seat and therefore technically going backwards, or because I like to see out of the windows at where I'm going when I travel, this particular trip was hard work. Generally, I don't get travel-sick, never before on an ambulance; it might have been provoked partly by the fact I'd had absolutely no sleep before the 12-hour night shift, so by the time I'd see my bed next, I would have been awake for 26 hours (this is where all the other frontline staff reading this will moan and groan that I've got it easy…)

The heating in an ambulance is usually set to somewhere around 'surface of the sun' and hopping in and out between that and minus five, allows no adjustment period at all. You just get used to being frozen (although paramedic jackets are quite toasty) and you're back in the sauna. Returning from an inter-county hospital transfer and driving 60 miles back at who knows what hour in the morning, with the regularly intermittent flash as each streetlight illuminated the mobile emergency room, my colleague realised I'd become very quiet. He saw the ashen colour my face was going and pulled me up front at the next service station. I didn't need telling twice. I think part of it was because he didn't want to have to scrub out the back of the truck after I'd projectile vomited all over it.

NHS Discounts

You only have to look on social media and there's a 'well done' post for this coffee shop or that takeaway because they've given ambulance personnel their lunch for free to say thank you. I love to read that. I love to read that people behind them in the queue have paid for their orders or that they've been allowed to skip the queue altogether. Ambulance personnel especially never really know when their meal break will be, and there's always so much negative publicity around emergency service response times, so small recognitions like this really remind me how much gratitude the majority of the public have. I think it's fantastic and if I was ever to work in a tea shop or whatever (because I really don't think I will be on my knees bandaging bilateral leg ulcers when I'm 70), that's probably where all of my pension would go – reimbursing the business for all the free stuff I've given out to the emergency services.

It's always lovely to find that companies recognise the hard work of the health service and offer NHS discounts. Some of these can be quite substantial and the range of businesses that offer them, from retail to travel companies, beauty treatments to airport parking, can be surprising sometimes. I love finding a bargain anyway, then to find out it offers up to 60% off for NHS staff really makes my day, especially since I can't claim student poverty anymore. I've recently discovered that a usually quite pricey spa and salon I like, offers 25% off for NHS staff, allowing me to afford a more regular spot of pampering as a pay day treat. Not everywhere advertises the fact they do this though, so for future reference, there's no harm in asking. In fact, some places offer more of a discount than I got as a student, and now I've got to be an adult and do adult-y things like pay for home insurance and switch energy providers every so often, the discounts are much more useful...

Into the Big Wide World

So there I was, stood in my uniform with my identity badge saying 'Community Staff Nurse'. I would be supernumerary for a little while, to settle in to the job, and to take advantage of the extra support I would get as a newly qualified nurse. I had lots of role-specific training coming up, my preceptorship, as well as meeting my new colleagues and patients. It felt like the first day of school but by the fifth week of being supernumerary, I was chomping at the bit to be let loose on my own. I actually had to beg my manager to let me out. Personally for me, I felt like I was still in a student comfort zone and as I was now registered, I didn't want to be so wrapped up in cotton wool. Looking back, I gave myself a baptism of fire and although it worked out well overall, I should have perhaps taken the molly-coddling for a bit longer and taken full advantage before being sucked into the pressures of a short-staffed team full to the brim with patients who need this that and the other.

A month after I was given free reign over my own set of patients, the death toll remained at zero and it felt like I'd been a registered nurse for years. I was starting to develop strong friendships with co-workers, friendships that have persisted even though we no longer work together, and within a few short months I also became an Infection Prevention and Control Link Nurse for the team. Even though I had to take a step back for a little while a few months in, starting my nursing career in a district nursing team was the best decision I'd made, considering I had no idea what area I wanted to work in.

Hello life as a community nurse.

What Time Are You Coming?

One of the primary factors in deciding eligibility for DN visits, is that the patient is unable to get to their GP surgery to see the Practice Nurse (PN). If you are not housebound (this does not include the fact that it might well be easier for us to come to you), generally you do not fit the criteria for home visits from the District Nursing Team (DNT). This may be temporary or permanent, and discharging you to the practice nurse may be one step in your recovery; it means your mobility and independence is improving.

As you are housebound (because why else would you be referred to the DNT), aside from situations such as hospital appointments, funerals, the surgery being close for weekends and bank holidays and other such one off events, we assume you will be at home all day. So please don't ask us what time we're coming because you're going shopping/playing bowls/walking your neighbour's goldfish. We don't know. If you want a specific time to receive nursing care that fits in with your busy schedule, the practice nurse at your surgery can arrange that for you. If you do have a hospital appointment or require daily care on weekends when the surgeries are closed, we will be more than happy to accommodate however, we still can't give you a definite time. All we can do is agree we will visit in the morning or afternoon, or reschedule for another day if appropriate. If a patient's needs mean we have to visit when care staff are present, we will agree a time that suits all parties

– we don't want to make life difficult for ourselves or others. If a patient lives next door to someone we have to visit at 11am, common sense puts the two visits together, but this depends on clinical need and the staff skill set we have available on that day.

We are doing our best working with the system so please don't be upset with us that we can't tell you when we're coming. Understandably, people can settle, plan their day and arrange visiting times with friends if they know a time to expect the nurse. As someone who has had to stay in all day waiting for a delivery that could be between 8am and 6pm (which turned out to be 5:55pm) I can understand how restless it leaves you, wondering if the ten minutes you decide to take a shower or eat a meal will be the ten minutes the doorbell will ring.

Believe me, we would love to be able to give you a time but even if we could, due to urgent calls and outside influences, we might have to change that time on a daily basis. Generally, in my day to day duties, I advise it could be anytime between 9am and 4pm, because of the insulin visits at either end of the shift, but the day service is actually available for visits between 8am and 6pm. Most patients are fully cooperative and quite pleasant about it. Requesting a visit after 9:30am because you have to drop the kids off at school, or letting it slip that your husband with the car doesn't get home from work until 2pm will earn you a little less sympathy from me. If I spend half an hour listening to all the reasons your social life is better than mine, don't be surprised if I discharge you to the practice nurse.

Just a Carer

Community nurses work alongside care staff to provide good quality care for our patients, whether they work in a care home or for a company that carries out home visits as part of a social services provision. Yes, I am **the** nurse and you're not. Yes, I deal with things that you're not qualified to do. I have earned my title and you don't have one. But please please please, stop referring to yourself as 'just a carer'. Give me a pound every time I've heard that since qualifying and it could have paid for my first year's registration fee.

I am no stranger to self-doubt and worrying that I'm not doing a good enough job, but it is seriously a pet hate when care staff feel that they have nothing of value to contribute the minute a nurse's uniform walks through the door. Some carers visibly stiffen and all of a sudden behave as though the CQC have just walked in. If I ask a question, I'm not about to give you a telling off (unless you deserve it), I'm merely asking a question. Have faith in yourselves.

Sadly, there are carers who seem to simply put in their hours and go home, but these are a minority and you can guarantee I will pull them up about it if it affects my patient's wellbeing. I might be the trained nurse, but I visit the patient for a short amount of time once a day or even once a week. You are with the patient much more often and, in regards to care home staff who are the biggest culprits for saying they're just carers, 24/7. I am asking you about the patient because you know so much about them that can help me in my assessments, particularly when the patient is unable to tell me themselves. If I ask how a patient has been since I last visited, please don't say "I don't know, I'm just the carer". Even if all you can say is that you haven't noticed anything different in appetite or general mood, I can begin to base my assessment around this. If you say Mr G has been a bit more short-tempered with you than usual (and I have no reason to agree with him), it allows me to be alert to the possibility that something else might be going on, such as an infection or deterioration in mental health. What you as a carer can tell me is invaluable information, just as what I can advise you will enable you to provide individualised, consistent care. We are a team.

I've been on both sides; I've worked as a care assistant for twelve years, in care homes and in hospitals, before qualifying as a nurse. On the occasions it's happened, usually by someone with a superiority complex, being described as 'just a carer' is incredibly patronising. It made me feel two inches tall when in fact, if you asked, I could tell you that Mrs S is incontinent not because she's lazy, but because she is so scared of falling again that she daren't walk to the toilet on her own and is too proud to ask for help. I could tell you that Mr C isn't refusing to go into hospital because he is being difficult or because of his dementia, but because he is terrified that, just like his wife of 65 years, he won't come home again.

We build a strong rapport with those we look after, sometimes being preferred to the patient's own family. We know how they have their tea, whether they like to brush their teeth before or after breakfast, and what time in the afternoon they start getting too tired to be cooperative. I appeal to all registered healthcare staff, please don't dismiss a carer because they don't have a degree or because they might get paid half of what you do. Many have heard the saying 'behind every good doctor is a great nurse'; I extend that and add 'behind every great nurse is a fabulous healthcare'. Good care staff are worth their weight in gold because they know the patient far more than we could ever comprehend.

Just a Carer Pt 2

On the other side, sometimes there is a need for us to refer to you as 'just the carer'. Because some bright spark decided it would be a good idea to use the same uniform as nurses, especially in the community. This causes confusion and to be honest, annoys me.

In the hospital I worked at, all levels of clinical staff were differentiated by their uniforms. There is currently a push for theatre staff to wear caps which state their job role (because you don't know who's who when everyone is in scrubs) and in the latest heatwave, local hospital staff were complaining that they weren't allowed to wear lighter, cooler scrubs on shift, but it's because it doesn't allow instant recognition of their role. I understand this, in a world where you can't wear lanyards or badges and this that and the other. I've had a paramedic start handing over a patient to me as though I were a doctor in A&E majors one night because I was wearing scrubs instead of my normal HCA uniform (which by now hung worse on me than a bedsheet).

Between the DNT, different levels of staff wear different uniforms. It's important. I'm proud of my uniform, quite defensive of what it stands for and if there's one thing I will iron to within an inch of its life, it's my uniform. So when patients confuse us for carers because they wear the same one, it gets on my nerves.

I've seen patients, introduced myself as the nurse, and carried out whatever I was there for. At the end of my visit, I'm asked what else am I going to do. Meaning hang out the washing, prepare dinner etc. Even though I've explained I'm the nurse, the patient thought I was the carer because of the uniform. Now, if the patient thinks I'm the carer, do they think the carer is the nurse? Some carers tell patients inaccurate information thinking they're doing the right thing. This can lead to misleading information and complaints because "the other nurse said..." and as the patient has become quite fond of the care staff from where the information came from, it can sometimes be quite a challenge to make them realise that actually, the advice given isn't correct and is potentially causing more harm than good. This is where, if we need to get a bit tougher, we will say that the carer is just a carer. We don't say it lightly but when incorrect advice is becoming detrimental to the care we are providing, when a patient refuses to understand how in the world their 'lovely carer' could possibly be wrong, we have no other choice.

Nobody confuses the greens of the ambulance service or police uniform so why should community nursing be any different? Smart as they are, I don't think care companies need to provide NHS type tunics. A polo shirt would do (as porters in hospitals wear, to differentiate them from clinical staff). Patients and their families can be easily confused, and it's no wonder where conflicting information comes from.

Skin Tears Galore

For some reason, there are certain days (usually weekends) when there is an influx of SOS calls for new patients with skin tears. Skin tears in the elderly can be caused by the most minor of trauma; slight injuries that would barely bruise us can cause devastating tears in frail people, owing to the fragile tissue-like nature of the skin as it ages. I've been called to skin tears the size of the palm of my hand on patients not much bigger than your average seven-year-old. Shark bites we affectionately call them.

I do love a good skin tear – it's almost like creating a piece of artwork, rehydrating the skin flap and securing the edges back together to encourage healthy wound healing with minimal lasting damage. However, what I don't love, is when the skin tear has gone unreported/unnoticed and by the time I get there, the flap of tissue has died, the wound bed has become unhealthy and there is inevitably going to be a long-term complication left behind. Prompt treatment of skin tears, especially on the lower legs, is essential to avoid potentially weeks of treatment and even the development of ulcers, leading the patient needing to be in compression therapy for months.

Frustratingly, the majority of skin tear SOS calls come from care homes. Obvious really, seeing as that's where the highest concentration of elderly and frail people is. Also frustratingly, many care homes also provide for nursing care as well as residential, meaning they have a registered nurse on the premises. I am not in the habit of turning down first aid to those who need it because of funding conflicts. I don't understand why nursing staff and even senior care staff, cannot be educated by the DNT to provide basic first aid care such as this. For the spectacular skin tears as described above, by all means call us and we will be there as soon as we can. But the majority of 'SOS' calls are for wounds so relatively insignificant that, when asked if they would personally put a plaster on it, the carer has replied "no I wouldn't". And yet, we're called out, having more than likely had to delay another visit until the following day, to attend.

I completely understand that care staff are not trained nurses, but neither are our HCAs. Is basic first aid not a staff requirement in care homes? At every care home I worked at in my younger years, it was a mandatory requirement as part of the induction training. A single scuff on a patient not previously on our caseload not only entails wound assessment, but also photographs, malnutrition scoring, pressure risk assessment and incident reporting, equipment ordering, all of which can equal at least two hours of administration on top of the actual wound care. I know many care staff who wouldn't have called us out but felt they had no other choice, even when there's a trained nurse at the other end of the corridor.

This is also true of insulin administration in care homes. When there's a registered nurse employed in the same building, I can't get my head around why they can't administer insulin as part of their medication round, thus saving the DNT visiting twice or sometimes three times daily. Once again, it comes down to funding. Even though a suitably trained carer provides the medication for a resident in a home, sometimes at the same time the community nurse is present, they can't give insulin because that service comes out of a different budget (in my area anyway – I can't speak for other areas in the country). Surely, it would save a huge amount of government money if care staff were adequately trained to administer insulin. I understand concerns that it's a medication being injected into the body and it would open a new can of worms in case anything went wrong, but a large number of diabetics administer it themselves, and we educate and support friends and family to give an insulin shot and they aren't even carers, let alone registered professionals. Even our Band 3 HCAs are being trained to administer insulin and a neighbouring Trust allows family members to administer PRN medication in end of life patients. The mind boggles.

No Ambulances Available

Working as a team is vital in the NHS, regardless of which department you work for. I realised that especially on a New Year's Eve shift in the community. An SOS call came in for a skin tear (!) not from the patient but from the ambulance service. Being New Year's Eve, with possibly one of their busiest nights ahead, the patient's son had called for an ambulance after his elderly Mum had a fall which resulted in one of those whopping great big skin tears I'm such a fan of. No ambulances were available and sadly (although also, in some respects, rightly) she was not considered a priority call and could be waiting hours for an ambulance to take her to A&E, where she might wait even more hours to be seen. She was unable to travel to hospital herself so the call came from the ambulance service through to us, along with an apology. Direct calls from the emergency services such as this are quite unheard of.

I responded to this call immediately because as I've said, prompt treatment of skin tears is essential to reduce further complications, poor healing and unnecessary scarring. I was there within an hour of it happening. It was impressive as far as skin tears go, a good 10cm by 5cm on her lower arm and yet unbelievably, she denied any pain. After a good clean up, nearly a whole pack of adhesive stitches and a suitable dressing later, I came away feeling like a job well done. The wound healed beautifully, something which wouldn't have happened if she'd waited hours for treatment. After being patched up in A&E she would have been discharged to us for ongoing wound care anyway, so to step in and save the ambulance a trip and the lady a day at the hospital, it felt like a minor victory of sorts. I've also seen A&E nurses patch up skin tears and I have to say it, they're not as good at it as us, the community wound care champions who see them day in day out (we also know the long-term effects that **we** will have to deal with, so it is slightly for selfish reasons).

We try to reduce the burden of unnecessary calls to the ambulance service, and it's something in particular I work really hard to promote. Sometimes, obviously an ambulance is needed; we call them ourselves regularly for falls, head injuries, suspected sepsis etc. I take every chance to educate patients and carers about whether or not they should call an ambulance but I always reiterate, if you are that concerned, best to call an ambulance and not need it than to wait. At the end of the day, it's not my place to gauge the concern of the patient/relative and decide they absolutely do not need the emergency services.

I've come across mainly two types of people in this job: those who will call the emergency services for the silliest little thing (and at times, these reasons are insanely infuriating) and those who won't call an ambulance until we have to do it for them because they "don't want to make a fuss, they're so busy". There are those who realise the happy medium and it's this sense of awareness I continually try and promote. There are other services you could contact first if you're not sure whether something constitutes an emergency or not. I rapidly run out of patience with relatives who wait seven hours for an 'emergency ambulance' for their loved one who's hurt their leg and then proceed to moan about how long they've had to wait, when they have two cars sat on the driveway. Calling an ambulance and arriving at hospital with two escorts in green uniforms does not mean you will be seen any quicker.

I'm Scared of Getting Old

One thing I've noticed myself thinking about more and more in this job, is how fragile human mortality is. I am reminded daily what I (hopefully don't) have to look forward to. Okay, this is a very broad statement because in this job, there's not much need for me to see happy healthy people who are flourishing in their retirement years. I'd like to think I'll spend my 'old age' tending a beautifully immaculate garden, baking apple pies for the grandkids and enjoying long lazy countryside summers with my husband. I try and avoid thinking about any other alternative than that.

Some patients do exactly that until they are too tired to carry on; they simply fall asleep. Others, sadly don't. I spent some time with the specialist palliative care nurse when I was in my supernumerary period and I honestly don't know how they can do that job all day every day. We provide palliative support for patients and those visits can be tough enough, but to deal with complex cases for the whole of your job, it must be so emotionally draining. Massive respect for them.

Some patients have been pleasantly confused; don't know what they've had for breakfast but are quite happy and full of conversation (even if it does consist of the same three questions with a bit of random chit chat thrown in). Some patients die at 105 in their own homes, surrounded by grandchildren and great-grandchildren and a

Yorkshire Terrier called Lucky. Some I have to double check their date of birth (and where they buy their anti-wrinkle cream) when they tell me they're 92 and have cut their arm whilst gardening. It's those patients that I want to be like when I'm older. Those patients really lift my day.

Other days, I've come away from patients who don't know their own name let alone recognise anyone else's because of dementia, who live alone with no friends or family nearby to spend Christmas with, and people who are so frail at the end of life, they literally look like a skeleton in a dress. It's frightening. Some days I've had to pull the car over and take ten minutes just to rebalance and admittedly, have a little cry, because I'd be a nervous wreck otherwise. This job really reminds you how not invincible we are, even though we may feel it in our teens, our twenties, thirties etc. It's saddening that sometimes the scariest thing is not that we could be hit by that bus tomorrow, but that we may end up in one of those situations, losing our friends, families, identities. It scares the hell out of me.

Why Aren't You Married?

I have to say it, some of my patients don't half give me a complex some days. I'm not sure why it's one of the first questions I'm asked but it comes up far too often for my liking really. People are either really nosy or it's just one of those 'safe' questions along with 'do you live around here?' Sort of like when you get a drunken taxi home after a messy night out. It's almost a form of British Tourette's; you just can't help but ask the same two questions:

"Have you been busy?"

"What time do you finish?" (Which I also get at work).

Nobody in the history of drunken taxis home has ever actually cared whether the driver has been busy or not, or what time they finish, but it seems to be a very British, very typical thing to do, and almost like an unwritten law along with apologising when someone else bumps into **you**.

When I reply no I'm not married and get asked why not, it always seems as though simply saying 'because I'm just not' isn't a good enough response. I suppose to the majority of our patients who are over a certain age, perhaps being the wrong side of 29 and not married is one of the worst things that could happen to a young woman. But times have changed and it's not an expectation anymore, it's a choice.

So, I'm currently working my way through a list to see which one will satisfy the interrogator:

- "Nearly" - (but this will lead to a tonne of further questions and I'm in danger of being tied to a chair and having a torch shone in my eyes).
- "I'm still waiting" - (in a tone not sounding too much like I spend every weekend hunting for Mr Right).
- "I can't decide which one to say yes to" - (maybe giving me a reputation I don't particularly want preceding me).
- "I don't see the point" - (possibly offensive to someone who has been married for half a century).
- "I don't know" - (does this imply there's something wrong with me?).
- "Some days I can barely look after myself let alone a husband" - (which naturally instils faith in the care you're about to provide).

For most patients, I've settled at the moment on just 'not yet' and quickly changing the subject before I start being questioned on every aspect of my love life. I haven't technically lied and they can interpret that as they will. Aside from one very charming gentleman who insists that the second I get married I'll lose my looks and my teeth (?) everyone seems to wonder why I'm still a 'maid' and it's quite honestly, a question I'm getting sick of answering. I feel like my opening greeting should be to introduce myself, say I'm not married and no I don't have children, what can I help you with today.

One lady (absolutely bonkers but the sweetest woman you'll ever meet) looked at me as though I'd just told her I've murdered her postman when I said I wasn't married. "But you've got a baby?!" she screamed at me. Now, the last time I checked, no I didn't have a baby, and I later found out that she was confusing me with another nurse who apparently looks just like me (the only similarity this other nurse and I share is that we both have brown hair). I'm curious to know where the conversation will lead when one day I do say "yes I am married". Will I then be interrogated about why I don't have children yet? Maybe I should add that response to the list as a kind of social experiment?

Bigger Picture

Nursing care is a holistic process – even in emergency care, you always have to be alert to the possibility of other things going on aside from the focus of your treatment. How much emphasis you put on certain aspects depends on your area of work, for example, if your leg is hanging off and you're bleeding to death, the circumstances surrounding your living conditions isn't going to be as high up on the list of priorities for the ED team. However, someone's living conditions will be important for the community nurse and it will be a big deal to the therapist who is going to help you gain the confidence after a fall. In the community, we are optimally placed to assess every aspect of your life and build a bigger picture so we can involve other teams if needed.

Sometimes in the community, calls come through with seemingly the simplest of reasons – 'red bottom', 'insulin while carer is away', something you might think is a straightforward VTD (visit, treat and discharge). This is where the importance of holistic assessments comes in. When that call comes in for a 'red bottom', they are never that simple. There is no such thing as 'having a quick check'. Holistic assessments and even just the general atmosphere of a visit can reveal so many things that suggest we could in fact, be visiting someone who is on the verge of a crisis. Our visit might have been the 'saved by the bell' moment before the patient is admitted to hospital, or in the worst case scenario, found dead three weeks later.

Some of the information we collect during our first visit to you (technically we have the first three visits to complete it – it allows for VTDs and capacity issues) include the following*:

*Tools and policies may be different for other areas of the country.

Photographs

Key in removing subjective information about wounds. It's so much easier to compare HD colour photographs than descriptions of colour and size. I'm sure infection control would have a field day if we were still using tracing paper on wounds!

Medication / Medical History

If you're taking blood thinners, steroids or immunosuppressant drugs, it allows a forecast of expected healing time. We can also tailor our treatments to address any contraindications – if you have a suspected DVT, aside from shipping you off to the nearest emergency department, we're not going to put compression bandaging around your leg to encourage it to bounce off up to your lungs. We will use iodine dressings with caution if you have a thyroid issue. If you have asthma, we won't suggest Ibuprofen to relieve pain.

MUST

Malnutrition Universal Screening Tool. This helps us

to determine whether you're at risk of malnutrition. This doesn't just mean you're too skinny; malnutrition can also occur in overweight people. In its simplest form, obesity in itself is malnutrition because the body is lacking proper nutrition (imagine someone who lives on a really unbalanced, greasy junk food diet). If you are at risk of malnutrition, you are at increased risk for the consequences of it.

Pressure Risk Assessment
Different areas use different tools – Norton, Braden, Waterlow. Basically, this tool assesses your risk of developing a pressure ulcer. Designed to be used alongside clinical judgement, it provides guidance in terms of mobility levels, sensory impairment, continence issues and other illnesses that could impact the risk, such as frailty and diabetes. Where this tool shows there is a risk present, the **SSKIN** bundle is also carried out:

SSKIN
This assesses whether appropriate measures are in place or what measures need to be in place to reduce the risk of further complications of pressure-induced damage. It includes skin checks, pressure-relief equipment/regimen, requirement for continence assessments, and dietary supplementation.

Holistic
The holistic covers demographics, whether there are hearing/visual impairments, comorbidities, and many other things that people may wonder why we

need to know: aren't we only there to dress the sore on your leg? Why do we need to know your next of kin? In case we can't get hold of you and need to check you're okay. Why do we want to know your religion? So we don't inadvertently apply a dressing made from pork gelatine and assume it's okay with you. The questions asked (or interrogation as it sometimes feels like) also allows us to refer to other services if we feel you would benefit:

If the patient has fallen four times in the last six months, do they need a referral to the falls team and a medication review?

If someone's been struggling with mobility after a long period of illness, would they benefit from physiotherapy to build their muscle strength back up?

Would palliative patients benefit from equipment to help them move around their house and maintain independence? If so, we'll get in touch with the occupational therapists.

If we're concerned about a patient's ability to look after themselves with increasing illness, we might suggest a referral to social services to assess for a care package to help with daily activities such as washing and dressing. We can also suggest respite / day care so the main carer (who is usually the husband or wife) can rest and recover. You can't fill from an empty jug.

We can arrange further assessments for continence if the patient is having difficulties with elimination – struggling to get to the toilet in time is one of the main causes of falls in the home.

Sometimes we may be concerned about a patient's mental capacity (consent is a big deal in healthcare) or worried that they're at risk of deteriorating mental well-being. We can refer to the mental health team.

Sometimes, we're concerned about the environment, whether it's because the patient is a hoarder or smokes in bed (in which case we refer to the fire service) or because tensions between family members or other 'care provider issues' may put the patient at risk of abuse. We can then refer to the safeguarding team and social services.

As this list (and it's not a complete list) demonstrates, we can gain so much information which will enable us to get the best help available for patients – we don't throw our weight around about it though, we do work with them and respect their wishes if they feel they don't want input from another service just yet. This is quite common in palliative patients. The introduction of mobility equipment into their home reiterates the fact that they are deteriorating. Sometimes it's not unusual for patients to refuse referrals at first, and then change their mind.

There are times when we intervene at just the right point before the patient or their family hits crisis point. We work alongside a rapid intervention team that can swiftly put temporary care packages into place while social services sort out carers, and arrange respite care before the main carer becomes very unwell with the stress of it all. Knowing we can provide so much support if it's needed is one of the biggest reasons community nursing is so rewarding. Yes, we see some awful things and sometimes all we can do is conservatively manage, but other times, we can make such a difference to someone's life, that it reminds you of the reason you became a nurse.

Attacking from All Angles

When I first started the job, I became quite heavily involved with one particular patient. This lady (we'll call her Mrs B) had horrific ulceration of her lower leg. Lovely lady, could talk the hind legs off a donkey; she came across as one of those women who, back in the day, would know everybody down her street and would have very set family traditions like Fish and Chip Friday. She was a very complex case and within three visits I had arranged for nearly everyone to see her, becoming the lead nurse for her care (some patients respond better to a consistency of the faces they see – it's easier to make a breakthrough if you're the face they really open up to). Nurses had been seeing her for months but she had refused all other input – she was quite proud and a little bit stubborn.

She lived in a typical two up two down house, and survived on Lucozade and cigarettes. The house was cluttered but because of the pain caused the leg ulceration, the last thing she wanted to do, and could physically do, was clean. Also, because of the pain, she didn't go upstairs. Not just to bed, but not even the toilet either; she used a bucket in the living room, where she slept on the sofa.

Mrs B was a very proud lady, didn't have carers and refused the conversation to be assessed for them. She said she ate well but an inspection of her kitchen cupboards told a different story, and she was very upset that she could no longer do the things she used to do, not even catch the bus into town. Some people choose to live in a certain way and that's not our choice to make for them, but going by how she spoke to me, I wasn't satisfied that Mrs B was happy with her quality of life. She felt like she'd been "brushed under the carpet". I really got my teeth into this one.

It was a hard job getting through to Mrs B; she had a fantastic knack of changing the subject when I tried to mention the other services available. We also hit a bit of a brick wall with family members, who were verging on becoming a safeguarding concern. As Mrs B struggled to cook "decent homemade meals" as she once could, I suggested a meal delivery service that provided nutritious balanced meals and all she would have to do is heat it up. She was quite interested about this but never truly committed as family members told her it was too expensive.

I arranged for OT (Occupational Therapy) to assess her home for equipment such as a wheeled walker and stair rails to make it easier for Mrs B to get around the house, and to provide a commode so she didn't have to do her business in a bucket. I arranged for Physiotherapy to visit to encourage her to do some mobility and strength-building exercises. Mrs B agreed to have a lifeline pendant and key safe put in place (only after she fell in the garden on a winter's evening and was there for a few hours). The Community Matron visited with me to try and address the issues around non-compliance (if you tell me you've only had one cigarette three hours ago and yet I come out of your house smelling like I've been dipped in an ashtray, forgive me if I don't believe you). A social worker came with me to discuss whether Mrs B may be better off moving to a one-level warden-supervised housing development where she could be prompted to take her medication properly and there would be 24/7 support should she need it, as well as other residents; Mrs B was far too chatty and sociable (albeit full of the proverbial) to live alone and spend her days watching TV.

Overall, aside from the frequent stumbling blocks, particularly involving Mrs B's family members worrying about how she was considering spending her **own** money (in my opinion, £50 a week to know my mother/grandmother is eating 2-3 nutritious, homemade meals per day is not something I would even have to spend time thinking about), we really started making headway with her.

I felt almost crushed when I returned from a week's annual leave to find out she'd been admitted to hospital, presumably with severe infection from her leg ulceration. Mrs B was in hospital for weeks and was discharged to a nursing home. It took a lot of persuasion from colleagues that I did what I could for her. I kept thinking to myself, what had I missed? Perhaps, if all of that intervention had been put in place sooner, the outcome may have been different? But then maybe not.

Aside from the importance of the holistic assessment, this care really utilised some of the key members of our multi-disciplinary team in the community, illustrating that effective cooperation amongst each team is how we can provide quality care for patients. Although Mrs B ended up in a nursing home, we had all worked together and were making good progress with her. I truly believe that had infection not hospitalised her, we would have managed to at least improve her quality of living, mental well-being and restored some independence, which indirectly may have eventually enabled the wound to heal.

What Do Carers Do These Days?

You will never catch me putting care assistants down, they are fantastic. I even make a mental note of the names of carers I come across who are exceptional – the internal monologue usually chats away to itself, "she's good", "finally someone who knows something without saying they're just a carer", "oh yes, they're on top of things".

However, I have noticed lately that care companies (those who send carers to patient's homes however many times a day for personal and domestic care) have newfound policies that mean they can't do this that and the other. All of a sudden, carers aren't allowed to change catheter leg bags once a week because of the risk of infection – what?! Surely that goes hand in hand with personal care? Changing a leg bag once a week is encouraging infection no more than flipping the valve and emptying the bag several times a day. Both break the closed system. The risk of infection is higher when the bag isn't changed as it's meant to be. The bag can be so old it's discoloured and full of sludge but please, don't replace it with a new one because it might cause an infection.

My HCA reported today that a patient had his catheter pipe twisted twice around his underwear and the patient's wife said the carer's won't touch it because "it's the district nurse's job". **Really?!** First, how on earth has it become twisted around his underwear – this would only happen if we did it on purpose when we inserted the catheter or it wasn't secured to the leg properly. Second, have they honestly just left a patient with his pants around his knees because it's wrapped around his catheter? How have they washed him properly? I think to save argument, some of the DNT would have straightened it out whilst there and seethed to themselves in the car afterwards. Luckily for the patient but unluckily for the care staff, my HCA is much more assertive; he went ballistic and demanded that the relative called the care company and got them back to sort it out. It's okay the DNT doing it this time, but what about tomorrow? We can't run the risk of the patient not receiving the personal care he needs because care companies aren't doing various different tasks that they are very capable of doing. I had a similar conversation with a relative who refused to be taught how to change a leg bag because "the doctor said it's a medical procedure and the district nurses need to do it". No. We would be so inundated with catheter leg bag changes that we wouldn't get anything else done.

Carers won't apply a new dressing if one has fallen off. If the dressing is complex or the wound is a bit complicated then fair enough, I understand, but what about when the dressing is basically like a plaster? Come on.

I've had a patient complaining that carers won't wash their leg because we had put Clinifast on it (similar to a Tubi-grip stocking) to stop pressure-relieving boots rubbing on their skin. This poor (bedridden) lady had gone without having her legs washed for weeks because the carers wouldn't touch the 'dressing'. My response? (Besides muttering some very grown up language to myself) – "take it off, cut the toes off a sock and put that on". Same job, but because it's a sock, now they can touch it. Honestly. Again, it's become defensive practice – they wouldn't take their child back to the doctor if a plaster on a grazed knee fell off, but because it's a working relationship, the rules and willingness changes.

On a positive note though, some care home staff are quite good at using their common sense when dressings fall off. There are some people I'm sure that panic, run around like headless chickens and threaten to quit if the district nurse doesn't come out right this second and replace it! But then some will just put on what fell off (new one obviously), and call us to let us know. We'll make a plan to get there when we can (if it's a care home, it's usually the same day) but at least the wound is covered for now. These are the carers I take note of.

Some carers now aren't allowed to prompt a patient to administer their own insulin because "it's medication". So are their morning tablets and you're allowed to prompt people to take them? If they need prompting, chances are you only have to say the word 'insulin' loud enough so they can hear you. Hell, you could even write it on a piece of paper and wave it in front of their face and not have to utter a single word! When was that banned? Madness. The frustrating thing is, it's not the carers refusing. It's the care company managers who have changed their policies – to us, it just seems they are charging the same for doing as little as possible, after all, what are district nurses for? The carers are usually more than happy to do these things. Again, politics and management gone mad.

The Strength of the Dying

One area of my job that I particularly enjoy, is palliative care. It's emotionally draining sometimes but I feel privileged that I will play a role in ensuring somebody will die with dignity. When someone reaches that stage where they need regular medication to keep them pain-free during their last days, although the patient remains the number one priority, it's somewhat humbling to be in a position where the family almost rely on you for support. You not only provide care for the patient, but also emotional care for the relatives.

Where patients begin to require PRN medication (an injection of drugs to ease symptoms as and when needed, when they're no longer able to take medication by mouth), the atmosphere can become very tense very quickly. Previously positive relatives can become quite distressed at the realisation that their loved one is nearing the end of their life, and understandably so. When the same nurse visits for several PRN calls and replenishment of syringe drivers (changed every 24 hours), it can be most beneficial for the families and very rewarding for the nurse to be able to provide almost continuous support for patients and their families at their most vulnerable time.

A particularly fond memory of providing palliative care that stands out for me is a lady in a care home who, for the most part of the day, was asleep. Once

PRN medications were started, she was needing visits roughly every 5-6 hours for repeat doses. Where the need for PRNs hits four in a 24 hour period (according to local policy), we consider the use of a syringe driver, which is a pump that continuously delivers a very low, very slow dose of the PRN medication over time to maintain adequate symptom control. This lady, Mrs A, had been on our caseload for some time before we started providing care for her in her final stages, so I knew her quite well. From Friday to Sunday, I visited several times for PRNs, arranged a syringe driver (which I finally got sorted at 20:50 on the Saturday night, four hours after my shift ended) and essentially became the named nurse for this lady over the weekend. But, true to her character, Mrs A made me work hard to keep her pain free and comfortable in her last days. Stubborn right to the end will be my fondest memory of her.

When the need for PRN medication becomes more frequent, and to enable attachment of a syringe driver, instead of repeatedly stabbing someone with a needle all the time, we insert a cannula which can remain in place for up to five days. Mrs A got through four cannulas that weekend. Within thirty minutes, every time I inserted one and administered medication, she'd pulled it out (conveniently waiting until I'd left the car park). Whenever I visited, she appeared to be more or less asleep. This is where we rely on care staff and relatives to let us know when the patient is agitated compared to their 'usual' self. They will be aware of the minor changes in condition that, because we're not there all the time, we wouldn't otherwise pick up on.

Where patients are little and frail, they don't usually have a lot of squidge (official medical term for fat) so sites to insert the cannula can be limited. I put one in her thigh (my number one go-to area usually), that was pulled out. I put one in just above her buttock, that was out. By now, with her need for PRNs so often, I was ready to arrange the syringe driver however, these are connected to the cannula. If she wouldn't keep the cannula in, a syringe driver would be ineffective (except maybe to her pillow). As a last resort I inserted one between her shoulder blades. Surely she couldn't yank that one out? How wrong was I. Twenty minutes after I'd left, it was out. I was beginning to think I was going crazy. Had I even inserted it? This poor 90-something year old woman couldn't even turn herself over, how on earth had she reached around and pulled it out of her back? Even to her death, Mrs A was as stubborn as ever; she had a tendency to refuse treatment and clearly this wasn't changing anytime soon. Unfortunately, she wasn't able to tell me she didn't want the syringe driver so I was acting in her best interests to reduce her pain and agitation.

Finally, after the fourth cannula was inserted lower down her back, two days after the first, it stayed in and the syringe driver was connected. Whether that's because she had deteriorated and lost her gymnastic flexibility or because she realised I wasn't going to give up easily I'm not sure, but either way, it was a success. Mrs A passed away peacefully with her family around her only a couple of days later.

Palliative support truly humbles me, although it can sometimes feel like you're on stage when you have ten pairs of eyes watching you draw up the controlled drugs, and then double check them, and check them again. In hospitals, controlled drugs are checked and signed for by two registered nurses. In the community, we're on our own. There is nobody to second-check, it is completely and solely down to us to get it right so it's essential that our drug calculation skills are up to scratch.

I love to see lots of family members; far too many die alone. In palliative care, for a few hours, you as a nurse become part of that family and it's one of the most rewarding parts of the job. Where death is expected and in some way controlled, you have played a part in making sure that the lasting memory the family have of their loved one is that they died peacefully and pain free. Everyone has different wants and needs in life; to find love, to have a nice house, to retire wealthy, but I'm sure we can all agree that, when it comes to the end, that's the one wish we all have in common.

Pressure Damage Vs Moisture Damage

Perhaps one of the most common things we see in the community, is pressure damage. Pressure ulcers, bedsores, decubitus ulcers, all the same name for damage caused by being in one position for so long that the underlying tissues become starved of oxygen and begin to break down. Damage can range from stage 1 (reddened skin that doesn't go white and back to pink when pressed, 'non-blanching') through to stage 4. SDTIs (Suspected Deep Tissue Injury) look like dark purple bruises and they can either resolve or break down revealing an instant stage 4 (fat and bone involvement and a rancid smell).

A large part of our workload is getting appropriate equipment and advice in place before pressure damage occurs. This doesn't come without its own barriers; issues with regular repositioning can lead to further breakdown or prevent healing, smoking in bed can restrict the choice of pressure-relief kit we can provide, and infection can halt healing for a long time. Pressure ulcers can be small, like the size of a matchstick head on the outside of a bony ankle, or they can be extensive and large enough to fit your fist into (and on some occasions, I've had to do just that).

Despite the prevalence of pressure-induced damage, it's nearly always preventable. Some patients refuse equipment to prevent damage, or don't use it correctly – I knew a lady once who refused an inflatable pressure-relief mattress because it would mean her cat couldn't sleep on the bed.

Someone else sat on a pressure-relief cushion but wedged two towels either side of it.

Some patients can't move themselves adequately or are unable to ask for help when they're getting sore because they can't feel it; here lies the importance of care staff routinely repositioning those at risk (every 2 hours during the day if possible) and us encouraging the patient to have a wander to the kitchen and back every so often (if they can). Some patients however, especially dying patients, are unfortunately inevitably going to break down as their frame becomes so frail. In these cases, repositioning isn't a priority for pressure area care, it's for comfort only – regular turning of a dying person can cause pain and be more distressing than beneficial for pressure relief.

Patients can develop pressure damage not only on their bums and heels (hot spots) but on their ears (from oxygen pipes), noses (from oxygen masks) and even the tips of their toes (from the sheets being tucked in too tightly). I've attended a patient who got pressure damage from her own body due to contractures. It doesn't take a poorly person's body much persuasion to develop a pressure sore but in most cases, they are entirely preventable by simple education of patients and staff.

Pressure ulcers can be mistaken for moisture lesions and vice versa. They sometimes occur together. Moisture lesions tend to be quite common in patients who are incontinent and first appear as superficial grazes on the skin. They are caused by the level of acidity of the skin being changed by urine/sweat/faeces, which leads to breakdown. This is the same mechanism of injury that causes nappy rash in babies. Although they can be uncomfortable they can be healed quickly if caught soon enough; they are most easily prevented and healed by keeping the area clean and dry and applying a **thin** layer of barrier cream (not daubed on so thick you can take it off with a spoon).

In housebound patients who are able to mobilise independently, where pressure damage occurs, it's quite often alongside moisture issues. These patients tend to be non-compliant and non-hygienic. These are also the patients less likely to help themselves by doing simple things like having a wash. Apparently, being told "it's moisture caused by sweat" is a lot more offensive than "it's pressure because you sit on your arse all day".

As a student, I saw horrific moisture lesions that needless to say, resulted in safeguarding referrals. During a night shift on a medical ward, a patient was admitted and he had such extensive moisture lesions across his buttocks, they looked like a slab of raw meat. The skin had literally been stripped away. Such massive damage which was unlikely to heal given his comorbidities (I actually think he died shortly after admission), all down to being left in wet incontinence pads for too long.

Not all moisture lesions are on the bottom, some are under the breasts, in groin folds, and in neck folds (in contracted patients as well as obese patients). I've even seen moisture damage on the front of someone's legs because they refused home help and sat in leg bandaging soaked in urine and wound fluid for most hours of the day. I'm not sure what's worse here; having ulcers that have their own resident maggots (yes, this has happened) or sitting in p**s all day. Mind you, I suppose there could have been worse products of elimination to be sitting in all day (this too, has happened).

Work Me is a Little Bit Spoiled

Whilst I don't shout it from the rooftops that I'm a nurse, when I go about my work day obviously wearing my uniform, I have noticed that members of the general public are a lot nicer than perhaps they would normally be. I'm making this comparison purely on my own experience, but I have definitely noticed that people are more comfortable around my uniform.

In a world where people tend to keep themselves to themselves, and on the road it is now very much every man for himself. I have to admit, I do quite like the respect and acknowledgement that people have for the blues. Strangers are more likely to smile and say hello when I walk past, instead of merely glancing in my direction, eyes down (my smile is the same in and out of uniform so I'm pretty sure it's not me). I'm encouraged to queue-jump in shops (sometimes) and customers behind me have paid for my lunch as a gesture of thanks. I don't have to spend five minutes trying to pull out of a junction in my car when my uniform is visible, I'm waved out with minimal waiting (not by Audi drivers though, they have a reputation to uphold).

I've even had a rather irate gentleman banging on my car window before now, getting quite worked up that I 'park outside his house all day every day!' After I recovered from the mini heart-attack, I wound my window down and said "I can assure you I don't". As he started to argue with me, I subtly unzipped my fleece and the moment he saw my blue uniform, he apologised so profusely I wouldn't have been surprised if he had offered me his driveway to park on whenever I felt like it. I giggled to myself all day about that one. Being parked in one spot all day. Hilarious.

Self-Mummification

As a nurse, I tend to have a pretty strong stomach. I think nothing of discussing open wounds and bowel movements with patients. Sometimes I have to tone things down a bit before I say it. Blood doesn't bother me, vomit I'm not so keen on but I can deal with it. Generally, not much phases me, I've seen it all; prolapses of various organs (which are always at the bottom end of the body), amputations, childbirth, hernia surgery and post-mortems. I can deal with skin so dry it either flakes off in chunks the size of my thumbnail or creates a mini-snowstorm. I can deal with all the weird and not-so-wonderful smells (aided by an overpowering dab of Olbas oil under the nose, effectively paralysing my smell receptors). But, even though I've experienced it quite a few times, body parts waiting to self-amputate really turn my stomach.

When blood supply is so damaged that the finger/toe/foot has become necrotic (devitalised and not far from dead), sometimes a decision is made by the consultant/surgeon to allow the affected part to self-amputate. For the DNT, this basically means daily dressing changes until it falls off. Why don't they just surgically amputate I hear you ask. Well, in order for surgical wounds to heal, they need a nice healthy blood supply to deliver oxygen and nutrients to the site and remove waste products effectively. In these cases, the nice healthy blood supply isn't there, it's already compromised, that's why the wound has occurred in the first place.

Our responsibility is to continuously monitor the wound for signs of infection (even though the whole area might look like one big infection, it usually isn't), cleansed and redressed regularly to remove exudate (the gammy fluid that comes out of wounds) and manage odour (trust me, once you've smelled gangrenous tissue you'll never forget it). We also provide emotional support for the patient and their relatives who have to deal with this situation every day. Gradually, the affected body part becomes drier and drier (self-mummifies) and shrivels right up before it does eventually fall off. Wet necrosis has a very different smell to dry necrosis but both are equally as rank.

All nurses have things they don't like – I've known nurses who can't stand the sight of blood or saliva and I can't deal with false teeth – and although we have a little moan about it, we don't have to live with it like the patient does. If anything, nursing puts everyday whinges and complaints into perspective, something everyone at some point could do with remembering.

One day I'm sure I'm going to remove a dressing and there will be a toe in it. I'm not sure how I'm going to cope with that…

Gangrene Where?!

Although (I hope) surgeons weren't waiting for this body part to fall off by itself, I have dealt with a patient with gangrene of the penis. It was during my very first training placement and yes, we were dressing a penis every day that was affected by wet gangrene (the tissue isn't drying out, it's basically just rotting - we don't use the term gangrene these days – it's 'devitalisation').

I can't remember how this guy ended up with this issue although I do think there was an element of denial and poor hygiene involved. I hope he learned his lesson though – it might not have gone that far if he'd spoken out sooner. I don't even know the outcome – unsurprisingly though, there are limited treatments for the gangrene of the penis; maggot therapy (good luck trying to persuade any man to agree to that), amputation, restoration of blood flow (not as simple as it sounds) or reconstructive surgery. All options that don't sound too appealing when you're a man and it's your nether regions.

I'm Not Just a Nurse

I am off duty today. Whilst I love my job and it's my nature to care and give advice, when I'm not at work, please don't make me be at work. Yes, I am a nurse but I don't know everything and no I don't want to look at it. In order to maintain that ever-important work-life balance, I need to restrict my work mode to 37.5 hours per week as much as possible.

Let me make it clear now that I don't mean if somebody collapses in front of me on the street I'm going to cross the road and pretend I didn't see it just because it's my day off. If I have CPD study that I need to do in order to maintain my registration, I will likely do that in my own time. Chances are, I may have already worked a few hours overtime this week tying up loose ends because I didn't get chance during my working day. I may already be working extra hours to help cover staffing issues.

When I finish work and come home, I would like to shed the work persona and just be me. I am a nurse but I am not **just** a nurse. I am also a reader, a writer, a music fan, an obsessive compulsive cleaner, a daydreamer. I don't mind giving the odd bit of advice here and there as long as it's within my professional scope of practice, but when I'm off duty, please be mindful that sometimes, I just want to sit in the garden with a book and a glass of wine, or talk to my friends about how good/crap the weather is. I want to watch rubbish on TV, I want to daydream about the places I want to travel. I do housework, I overindulge with friends at lunch, I go out walking with no clear end destination. I would like to do all of that without being asked about the insect bite or scratch that may or may not be getting infected. I may offer advice off my own back, but I don't want to have to provide a running commentary by text over why the doctors in the hospitals are doing this that and the other when you're already there, and in all honesty, I don't particularly care that your Aunt Mabel is going to have her ingrown toenails removed next week. Talk to me about something else.

I love my work and some days I feel I could rant and rave with the best of them about how sad/arduous/exciting my day has been (and some days, that's exactly what I need to do), but it's important that I am valued for who I am as my own person, and not made to feel like nursing is the be all and end all of my existence. I don't want to feel bad because I want to kick someone in the shins when they say "you're a nurse, you should know". I found out the hard way what it feels like when work takes over your life – it's detrimental to physical and mental well-being, and sooner or later it will affect your ability to do your job anyway. Downtime is important and that is the most important lesson I will teach any nursing student.

Less Than Desirable

It's a certainty, unless you work in some picture-perfect village straight out of the fifties where everyone has thatched-roofed houses, and a flowerpot left to wilt causes local uproar, you will visit some areas as a community nurse that make you lock your car doors and wipe your feet on your way out. Whether it's one particular house or a whole area, I've had days when I've seen where my visits are and my heart has sunk. Generally, (but not always) the patient is lovely, it's just their home/neighbourhood that makes me cringe. Sometimes both the patient and the neighbourhood give you that 'short-straw' feeling.

Shortly after starting, I was sent to a patient who lived down a very less than desirable road. In a pre-warning by my colleague, I was told to look like I know where I'm going, because the last nurse who went down there and drove up and down a few times because she couldn't find the residence, ended up with a brick through her car window. I had literally that week got myself a brand-spanking new SUV and was suddenly terrified for it. I decided to make my uniform as visible as possible and told my colleague to give me a safety phone call in 45 minutes. It was only recently I'd heard that the DNT no longer required a police escort to go to this particular area. The patient was a nice lady and I was delighted to find my car still had all four alloys when I finished the visit.

Another area I didn't like visiting was a block of flats in a bit of a crap area where we visited an intravenous drug user for leg ulcers. Very much the stereotypical 'council estate flats' that are perhaps depicted on rough television programmes set in East London around gangs and poverty. The stairwell had puddles of (going by the smell) urine every few feet, cigarette ends, empty cider bottles. The flat we visited often had a few people milling around who smelled strongly of alcohol and heroin (a smell I've developed a keen nose for, as I've said before) – we were always to visit in two's because of the potential risk to safety. I never had any issues with these people or this area, but I did feel intimidated sometimes – it's definitely a case of faking confidence even if, on the inside, you are sh***ing yourself a bit. Fake it until you make it.

Once I'd stepped over the car tyre in the hallway (?) the patient was okay too, really. He was always polite, even if some days he was less than chatty. On a methadone programme, it was unclear whether he was still actively taking heroin or it was just his friends. I always preferred to visit this patient last because I came out of that flat with my uniform stinking to high heaven of cannabis smoke, and my legs always ached because I certainly wasn't going to risk it and kneel on the floor while I redressed his legs. I still wondered why we visited him – he didn't live too far away from a clinic that would redress his leg ulcers and surely, this would have addressed the safety issue. He was able to go out every day to collect his methadone so I'm not 100% sure how he 'qualified' for DNT visits.

The rough areas are just part of the job, and sometimes you'd find an absolutely lovely house (spick and span and perfectly decorated) in a crap area, or an absolute shed of a house in what you'd think would be a nice area. I've been to one house where the decorators literally walked out in front of me, refusing to re-lay a carpet because of the state of the room it was to go down in. I didn't blame them one bit, I think I would have done the same thing had I been a carpet-fitter. Unfortunately, my job is one where you don't really have a choice to refuse to provide care based on the state of someone's house.

Packing Wounds

I hate packing wounds. There, I've said it. Not so much shallow ones that are near the point they don't need packing for much longer, but those ones that extend some 10cm+ inside the body. I do it professionally and I do it well, but there's something really disconcerting about probing dressing ribbons into a cavity in the body that you don't 100% know where it's going or how far.

As a student, I had to pack an abdominal wound and the patient decided it would be absolutely bloody hilarious to yell out as soon as I put the probe into the wound to measure its depth. I could have cried. I think that's the life-changing event that has made me hate packing wounds so much. That and the horrible sucking sound the dressing makes when you pull it out. I've had to pack plenty of abdominal wounds including dehisced Caesarean-section wounds (surgical wounds that have split apart), and I've also had to pack sacral pressure ulcers that are so deep you can see the bottom of the spine. You can imagine what my face looked like when the measuring probe hit that. The horrible sucking sound followed by the horrible grating sound and then, only audible in my head, the horrible retching sound of me throwing up in my mouth a little bit.

Catheters and Hot Weather

Hot weather guarantees two things – grumpy staff and blocked catheters. Patients don't drink nearly as much as they think they do, even though they tell you they drink plenty. I advise patients that they need to drink enough to keep the urine clear and straw-coloured. Some however, can't see all that well or don't monitor this as effectively as they should, resulting in catheters bypassing or blocking. This means many SOS calls with a four-hour window (if it's truly blocked and you're in pain, and not just because you know all the right words to say).

We 'troubleshoot' catheter issues first, asking questions including whether there's a likelihood of constipation, pain level, fluid intake etc. Experiencing pain in the abdomen puts the call higher up the urgency list (more likely to be a true blockage) and these calls can sometimes result in the need to send the patient to the nearest emergency department. When the bladder is so distended with urine that it causes pain, we don't like to drain it all in one go. It has to be controlled because if we drain too much too quickly (more than one litre as per local policy) it can cause fluid shock. Basically what happens here, is that the combination of pain and stimulation to the nerves from the distended bladder increases the blood pressure, so removing too much fluid before the body has time to adjust can drop the blood pressure a bit too quick. Emergency departments are better equipped than a single nurse on the road to deal with any potential complications from rapid drainage.

I carried out a TWOC (trial without catheter) the other day. When people have indwelling urinary catheters, sometimes you can't just take them out and away they go, especially if they've had it for a long time. Over time, through constant drainage (free-flow), the bladder loses its tone as it's not filling/emptying, filling/emptying, and so the urge to urinate disappears as the bladder isn't ever getting full enough to stimulate this. We move to a flip-flo system (a tap directly from the catheter instead of a bag) to restore this tone, and then remove the catheter in a morning to see whether the patient can urinate on their own. Ideally, the flip-flo valve has restored tone and the patient now feels the urge to urinate, so removing the catheter is just another 'part of the drainage system'.

This TWOC patient, let's call him Mr J, had a flip-flo valve and had been managing fine for years with it. Today was TWOC day so I removed the catheter in the morning and advised I'd return later that day to scan his bladder and see how he'd got on. I gave him advice on what to do during the day and told him the immediate outcome would either be that the catheter would stay out, or it would go back in. Just before I left for his visit that afternoon (after successfully TWOC-ing another patient), a DN contacted me to say the patient had called an ambulance in extreme pain and the ambulance service wanted to know how long I would be (hoping to avoid taking him to hospital – ambulance crews don't catheterise). The patient had called 999 because he misread the contact number for our emergency line and "thought it was someone's name" (?) so it's always worth double-checking patients can read any contact numbers back to you.

I got to the house as soon as I could, because even if I were exempt from speeding tickets, which I'm not and it's probably for the best, roadworks slowed me down at every turn. The ambulance was there with a very relieved paramedic, "Gosh, am I happy to see you" he sighed. I got a quick handover from the paramedic and entered the house. Mr J was hooked up to all the kit and complaining that he hasn't had a wee all day and he's in so much pain. I asked how much he'd drank (as we advise one litre – you won't output urine if there's no input) – four pints. Oh my god really? But now was not the time to tell him off for drinking **too much**.

I asked the paramedic if he minded waiting in case I couldn't re-catheterise and Mr J needed to be taken to hospital anyway. He was quite happy to hang about, so I set about re-catheterising this guy and hoped there wouldn't be any complications so close to the end of my shift. 500mls of urine drained off. Hmm. Paramedic's observations were stable and within range. Another 450mls drained. Obs still stable and within range. No more urine drained after that, pain ceased and Mr J felt much better. Total 950mls of urine drained in one go. Almost at the limit. I set the paramedic free and discussed ongoing care with Mr J. I don't think we'll be trying to TWOC this guy again – this was the fourth failed TWOC he'd had. The catheter was obviously acting as a stent for whatever blockage there was in the urethra that was causing the retention, and that would be for Urology to deal with. I still managed to finish my shift on time despite that drama, even though I went to the next four patients smelling strongly of cannabis and fighting the nausea that came with it (nothing to do with me, but the joys of attending visits on a very typical, poverty-stricken council estate).

TWOCs are hit and miss. Blocked catheters in hot weather are something we can predict with quite a bit of accuracy, but unfortunately people tend to leave it until they do have pain. Nurses could do with catheters in the summer months – we subconsciously restrict what we drink I think, to avoid being caught short needing a wee. The first rule of nursing is 'do as I say, not as I do'.

It's Okay, I've Called an Ambulance

Despite the pleas advertised on every bus stop poster and in every GP surgery, there are still some patients who misuse and abuse the services available to them. As a district nursing team, we have a four-hour window to respond to the most urgent SOS calls. Generally, as soon as we get requested to attend, it's the next visit we go to and this is usually within the hour. We make patients aware of this window both at the start of the episode of care and when we receive the call. Again, we can't promise times, but we will try and assist over the phone and advise on the best course of action until, if appropriate, a member of staff can attend 'as soon as possible'. If we think you need to call an ambulance instead of us, we will tell you there and then. So when you call an ambulance because we can't make it to you before you've even put the phone down, it does get our heckles up a bit. This is blatant abuse of already stretched services.

There seems to be an overwhelming misconception that once someone has called an ambulance, that ambulance is theirs, they will be taken to A&E and, because they arrived with the paramedics, they will be seen immediately. This is not true. I've stood as part of an ambulance crew at 4am in the corridor of an Emergency Department for 129 minutes before now and can vouch that, just because you arrive in an ambulance, it does not mean you automatically skip the waiting room and are seen as soon as you get there. This patient was quite unwell but there was simply nowhere to put him (he probably should have been in Resus). The pressures within the NHS mean this simply doesn't happen. The staff do their very best to meet government targets but as with any area of healthcare, prioritisation is a key skill. Effective use of the ambulance service is something I feel very strongly about, and people who think going to A&E because they can't get an appointment with their GP for three days is an acceptable alternative, really frustrate me.

When we accept your SOS call, we will get to you as soon as possible and try to keep you updated as to how long we will be. When we call to let patients know we're on our way after we've changed around our visits for the rest of the day, to then be told "it doesn't matter now, I've called an ambulance instead" is a waste of our time and a waste of emergency service time. If you ever see a nurse hanging up the phone and screaming into her steering wheel, it's probably just me, right after one of these calls.

There are occasions where a patient has deteriorated before we've managed to get there and these are the exceptions, but our triage team are well-placed to prioritise the severity of the issue. If you call in an SOS because your leg is wet, and another SOS comes in at the same time for pain relief injections for a dying patient, we will prioritise the dignity and physical well-being of the person who has days, if not hours, left to live. If you call in an SOS for a wet leg after we couldn't visit as planned yesterday because you'd gone out, and then call an ambulance because we now can't make to you until tomorrow, you've just contributed to the already full to the brim workload of the emergency services.

The ambulance service work on the same principle of prioritisation as we do, so if the ambulance is on its way to you for a leaky leg and they get a more urgent call, for example a cardiac arrest the other side of town, it doesn't matter whether they're two blocks away or pulling into your street, if they are the nearest crew, they're going to be diverted. You will have to wait. The crews don't like to leave patients waiting, and many a colleague has felt saddened when relatives rant on social media that their mum/dad/neighbour has had to lay on the floor for three hours before an ambulance arrived. However, the cardiac arrest the crew were diverted to wouldn't have survived the 3+ hours if they had gone to the leaking legs first.

Prioritisation isn't about saying one person is more important than another, it's about deciding which clinical need is more urgent, and which can afford to wait a little bit. I would like to think the majority of people would understand this and most do, however, the **emergency** ambulance service is there to look after us in situations that may be life-threatening. Let's use the service responsibly and look after them.

Entitlement

One thing I absolutely hate is people who behave like they're entitled to anything they ask for, simply because they pay tax and national insurance. Please, never ever say to me, "I pay your wages". The belief some patients have, that because **they** pay tax and insurance, this means they are effectively paying my wages, really winds me up. In my job, where the vast majority of patients are elderly/disabled/unemployed, in most cases I can guarantee I am paying more tax and national insurance than them so essentially, I am paying my own wages (if you want to think of it like that). Saying to clinical staff that you pay our wages is demeaning and belittling. It insinuates that you view us as your own personal professionals who should be doing whatever you ask. We will do what we've been trained to do (and pay an annual registration fee/union fee for the privilege, not to mention being thousands of pounds in student debt) and use our clinical knowledge. We're not in this profession to pacify patients and their relatives.

Yes, I understand how frustrating it can be to have worked all your life and now struggle with disability and retirement benefits due to various different criteria and rules that various governments (not me so please don't behave like it's personally my fault) have imposed. But I too have been paying contributions since I was legally ~~forced~~ able to and if we really want to be pedantically simplistic about it, chances are I'm paying for your healthcare rather than you paying my salary. Do I mention that when I come to put another £80+ of dressings on your wound? Nope. The system doesn't work like that. If you must, view national insurance like medical insurance. Feel safe in the knowledge that you have access to free healthcare whenever you need it, most of the time for free. Or, if you still insist you're paying my wages, please please please can I have a pay rise?

As a student I was carrying out admission paperwork for a gentleman who had returned from the Middle East quite unwell. "If I pay a bit more can I have a private room?" Some London hospitals, that might have been a feasible question, but not in a rural County hospital. He'd come in with potentially infectious gastric pathology so he was getting a 'private room' anyway….

A Multi-Nation Country

Quick note to add to the previous entry; as well as feigning deafness if you mention that you are responsible for my monthly salary, I will not engage in any form of conversation about how your taxes are paying for "all the immigrants". If it weren't for non-British born workers, the NHS would be even more up that creek than it is now.

One in every eight NHS workers isn't a UK National. It always strikes me as amusing when someone who claims that immigrants are the downfall of Britain, seem to conveniently forget this viewpoint when they treat themselves to Chinese takeaway, ordered via their Samsung Galaxy (Korean), delivered in a Peugeot (French), which they eat whilst watching American sitcoms on a Japanese TV, which sits atop a cabinet from Ikea.

Antibiotic Resistance

As an 'Antibiotic Guardian' I'm dedicated to challenging unnecessary use of antibiotics in a bid to reduce overuse and the increase of antibiotic resistance. Overuse 'as a precaution' leads to nasty bacteria becoming toughened to the medication and therefore the drug has less impact when it's needed. In the community, with wound infections and urinary tract infections (UTIs) being quite common, I've known patients to be on antibiotics for a long time and some seem to think antibiotics will solve everything.

It's quite frustrating when doctors seem to be able to look at wounds and prescribe antibiotics without waiting for the microbiology results. When a patient has a UTI and is symptomatic, antibiotics are prescribed until the sample results define the specific bacteria and allow for a more targeted treatment. With wound infections, you can't really do this. Sometimes there isn't any infection at all, sometimes the only patch you've swabbed happens to be the only area where the nasties aren't (this is why you need a good swab technique), some infections you know the cause of by colour and smell – Pseudomonas has a very distinct blue-green colour and an even more distinct smell.

Referral requests have come in along the lines of 'urine smells bad, needs antibiotics'. A) If you're clearly a doctor, why are you calling us and B) unless the patient has actual symptoms of an infection (confusion, fever etc.) antibiotics **shouldn't** be prescribed anyway. Some patients don't understand this and think we're denying them treatment, especially when they have a catheter and they think it smells bad/is cloudy/looks the wrong colour. We don't dipstick test urine for infection in patients with catheters – the test strip will inevitably light up like a Christmas tree due to colonisation (normal bug communities) along the catheter. Most chronic wounds are also colonised, and unless there is biofilm (quite often looks like a shiny slime covering the wound bed) preventing penetration, we would try treating with a topical antimicrobial dressing/cream first before shoving pills down your throat, which can wreak havoc on the rest of your body.

Some people are too eager to take antibiotics and eat them like Smarties but as soon as they feel better, they stop, leaving the course unfinished. Some patients have even told me they've just finished antibiotics last week, even though according to the system, this 'last week' was actually June two years ago. A patient told me at every single visit for two weeks that their gangrenous body part will be cured soon because they're taking antibiotics that cost £400+ for the course (heck!). I've also had people tell me they need antibiotics because they have the flu. No. Antibiotics can have incredible side effects so I don't know why people are so eager to take them. I was given two sets of pills once for a cat scratch. A. Cat. Scratch.

My cat was injured and in the struggle to sort him out, I got some cat blood in a new cat scratch. Working at a hospital, I thought I'd get myself down to minor injuries to be on the safe side because I wasn't completely sure of my tetanus vaccination status. Instead, I was told I was immune to tetanus because I had five shots as a child so I'm now immune for life (don't know how many I had, I can't remember) and was given two different sets of antibiotics 'just in case'. I absolutely did not collect that prescription and made the hospital aware of irresponsible prescribing. Sounds harsh but our health and our NHS needs protecting.

End of Shift SystmOne

Technology is rather amazing. When it works properly, in healthcare it really makes life easier. We can access test results, make referrals to other services, archive and organise relevant episodes of care so they can be seen at a quick glance. This, providing you've given consent for record sharing, means that when we outcome your visit on a Friday evening, your GP can see it immediately instead of waiting until Monday.

Community nursing teams are equipped with laptops which is an excellent development, meaning we don't risk losing/damaging the vast amounts of paperwork we would have to carry around every day for our patients. A patient I visited only last week commented that she left district nursing around the time laptops were being brought in and "it must make life so much easier". When everything works as it should, yes it does, right down to saving time fighting through traffic in the morning because we don't have to go to the office first to collect our lists. They're there on the laptop before I leave the comfort of my own home, allowing me to use my time more efficiently.

Technology does fail sometimes. In my case, it always seems to be at the end of my shift. I can work for eight hours and not have a problem. I can stay up to date with all of my documentation, referrals, emails and incident reports throughout the day, and go home with nothing outstanding. However, other days, the gremlins I appear to have residing in my computer always seem to know when I've been so busy I have to document two visits, catch up on work emails, record an incident form for a new pressure ulcer, and make a referral to safeguarding in the seven minutes before it's 'home-time'. Then they come out to play and it's guaranteed the system will freeze and not connect to the network. It is also guaranteed to start working as soon as I get home, adding another 90 minutes of administration before I am officially finished.

I've also taken to stocking disposable thermometer strips in my clinical bag in the car. My electronic thermometer doesn't respond well to what it considers extremes of temperature i.e. anything either side of 17-22 degrees celsius. Particularly annoying in winter, when the incidence of chest infections is starting to soar and at least 50% of my patients for the day complain of feeling unwell. Imagine having to give vital signs figures down the phone to a GP with that Monday morning feeling and explaining that you're unable to get an accurate temperature because the probe has thrown a hissy fit. The joys of modern day technology.

Non-Compliance

Nursing is a holistic process, especially in terms of wound care. It isn't just going in, doing the dressing change and leaving. Many things can affect wound healing – diet, ambient temperature, smoking status. It's incredibly frustrating when the patient smiles and nods and you know full well they're not going to listen to any of the advice you've just given them. My heart does sink ever so slightly when I visit patients whose legs have swollen up so much with excess fluid, that I can literally see beads of the stuff coming out of the skin while I apply new, clean, dry dressings. This can be quite a tricky condition to manage anyway but it's disheartening when I ask "do you elevate your legs when you sit?" and although the patient tells me they've literally had them up all day, they're dropped in it by the relative behind them who's shaking their head.

My team has seen great improvements in legs once the patient elevates their legs, with patients going from twice daily dressing changes to twice weekly – it stops gravity pulling the fluid into the feet, resulting in the grossly oedematous lower limbs we see regularly. This is a bit of an issue when patients don't sleep in bed at night for whatever reason. A reclining chair is better than nothing, but it doesn't beat the flatness that beds offer. We don't suggest it for the fun of it. Many times, simple wounds would heal beautifully if only the patient rested with their legs up – the care of the wound is not just the dressing.

Nobody would ever have to tell me twice to put my feet up!

It's also a little bit annoying when we're told, often after months of advising the patient that they need to get their legs up, that "they were much better in hospital". That couldn't possibly be because you were in bed with **your legs up** could it?! We try for months to manage wounds that won't heal because of fluid, and as soon as the patient ends up in hospital (usually from an infection in a non-healing leg wound), the hospital is bloody marvellous because their legs have shrunk to half the size. One week back at home and back to sleeping a chair and hey presto, massive legs again. Cue the 'you don't know what you're doing' speech. If only we could routinely send non-compliant patients with fluid in their legs to hospital every so often. They do as they're told there and stay in bed like good little patients.

Sometimes, a little threat of our own works wonders. A patient I'd been seeing for two months had grossly oedematous legs which had caused the skin to break down, leaving patches of superficial skin loss. These have the potential to develop into non-healing ulcers and I had the conversation over and over again about elevating his legs when he's sitting. Would he do it? Would he heck. Now it was summer, and my patience was wearing a little bit thin with being in and out of a hot car to hot house and back again all day, I tried the tough love approach. I held nothing back as I told him, "If you don't elevate your legs, you're going in bandages". Really, bandaging is the best thing anyway as it slightly compresses the leg, reducing the fluid retention over time and therefore reducing the risk of skin breakdown. However, in my experience, if people don't want to toe to knee bandaging (and most don't in thirty-degree heat), and if they consent just to pacify us, they will have the dressings off the minute you leave the house anyway.

This guy was elderly and having his umpteenth course of chemotherapy (which doesn't help with skin integrity) and I was quite blunt with him, advising that I didn't want to be swaddling him up in this heat, but I would at the next visit if he didn't elevate his legs. Three days later when I visited, he had his legs up on a footstool. His legs were dry, the skin loss had healed, and he was over the moon. I'm not usually one to say I told you so to patients, but I did say it to him. "Okay, you've proved me wrong" he muttered. Thank goodness for that, I was beginning to think my nursing degree didn't mean a thing.

I like to work with patients, not dictate to them – they respond better when they feel like they have some control. I agreed that I wouldn't put dressings on again so he could have a proper shower (which in itself can make the patient feel miles better in themselves) but only on the condition that he continued with the advice I had given him. I think he will end up in bandaging but I like to be optimistic and hope we're working towards the point where he will remain compliant before he does end up having his legs wrapped up like a Hallowe'en mummy.

The patient was discharged with dry healed legs and went a month before coming through on triage with 'wet legs'. The pause when I asked if he'd been elevating his legs told me everything I needed to know about his compliance.

Serves Me Right

I love the sense of humour of some patients, even when it is at my expense. When patients are a little more original in their jokes, and if I'm not likely to have heard the same joke four times already by Tuesday, I can have a good giggle with having the wool pulled over my eyes.

Not long after I started the job, maybe seven or eight weeks in, I went to see a patient with diabetic foot ulcers. Still a little wet behind the ears and asking for it really, I talked through the treatment plan with the patient and his wife, and had a full-blown conversation with guy, referring to his wife every so often. Didn't think anything of it.

The second time I visited, the visit was much the same as the first one; light conversation, discussion of treatment plans etc. I thought I was getting the hang of this community nursing lark. Then they both started laughing at me. Completely clueless, I asked what was funny, and the patient said, "she's not my wife, she's my sister". The little monkey had had me on for about an hour and a half in total. For someone who has a history of being quick to pull people up if something isn't right, he did very well to let me carry on this far! I laughed, I apologised, but afterwards in the solitude of my car, I felt a little embarrassed. Not because the joke was at my expense because it was quite funny, but because I shouldn't have assumed she was his wife. In a one-bedroom bungalow, there was no reason for me to think otherwise but that just goes to show, all is not always what it seems.

The patient still tries to have me on now, but I've become accustomed to the 'banter', it keeps me on my toes. Well played Mr F.

Inappropriate Referrals

Referrals into the DN team can come from almost anywhere. Hospitals refer to us to ensure seamless care after discharge, GPs refer to us after home visits, the therapy team, care staff, care homes and even the patients themselves can refer in. These referrals go through our triage team who action them – they are either accepted or (less commonly) rejected.

Sometimes hospitals refer with the request for daily visits. Unless it's for daily medication, those requests remain just that. Requests. Particularly for wound care, we will decide whether daily visits are required on our first visit. I have also seen referrals from a hospital for us to visit the patient **at the hospital**. Really? How about no.

I have yet to find out the reasoning behind these referral requests; part of me wonders if the staff have a bet going on who dares p**s off the community nurses, or if it's some kind of pledge activity to induct the new nurses to the team.

We follow up the requests of course, to make sure it's not crossed wires and they're actually making plans for once the patient is at home, but at least two referrals in four months came from a hospital unit while the patient was still there, with no definite discharge date. "There's nobody here to do it" will not get the referral approved. You are in a whole building just bursting at the seams with doctors and nurses. Well, okay, given today's staffing shortages in healthcare, maybe not bursting, but in emergencies when we can't catheterise patients and we send them to you because you can, sorry if we don't believe you when you say you can't provide catheter care on the ward.

Other inappropriate referrals that will lead to rejection including requesting Doppler scans for legs with no wounds (unfortunately my particular team aren't commissioned to provide that service – call us back when the untreated legs have developed ulcers) and requesting visits because there are no appointments with the practice nurse (harsh as it sounds, not our problem – they don't take our visits when we don't have capacity).

At one point, I also had a new GP trying his luck with "patient feeling sweaty and feverish, could do with a check over". Well then Dr Lots-to-learn-about-nurses, off you go. I believe that's why you're the doctor is it not? The rejections might go against working as a team to provide care in some respects, but we can't accommodate 'overflow' patients. We have enough of our own patients to see with limited staff and time, without taking on more because there's no staff or appointments elsewhere.

As a student I was quite naïve and wanted to help everyone everywhere regardless. Now, I'm more aware and more realistic of the limitations of the healthcare service. In my first year of training, I probably would have thought nothing of using ten £15 wound dressings per week. Now, unless there's clinical indication for a more expensive dressing, I'm more vigilant about choosing dressings based on efficacy **and** cost. I never thought that I would develop that thinking but it comes with experience. I'm not saying cheaper dressings can single-handedly resolve the NHS financial deficit, but every little helps.

Can You Come Later? I'm Going Out

I'm all for patients getting out and about if they can; we don't want you to be sat at home all day every day (and not just because then we can discharge you to the practice nurse). But when we arrive, having fought through traffic in between timed visits, please don't ask us if we can come back later as you're going shopping. For one, it makes us feel a little bad when we tell you, actually no Mavis we don't have time (we'd rather you just not be there at all when we arrive). Disproving huffs by relatives because we're making you late, aside from being rude, is somewhat distracting. Two, it can come across as slightly expectant of you, as though we are expected to fit into your life when it suits, as and when you say. We don't sit around waiting for our visit to you, we have plenty of other people that need seeing. We work for the NHS, not you personally, even though we will work as a team with you.

Either tell us you're not going to be in when we forward plan your visits (so we don't show up to an empty house) or just be in. After all, to need our services, you are meant to be housebound. If you can go shopping/to bingo/to see Uncle Tom every Tuesday morning, you can time that with a visit to your practice nurse. And if you call to ask what time we're coming because you're going to the doctors, guess what. Practice nurse.

A Million and One Key Codes

Key codes. For key safes or main doors, they're marvellous. When we can remember them. Most of the time, they're available on the system, which we nearly always forget to look for before we get to you, and when we realise you have a key safe, the computer decides to take a lifetime to wake up so we can get it (or your phone number so we can call you and ask what it is). My personal tricks include punching in the key code six times trying to get out of the care home and then spending five minutes searching round for a member of staff, to watch them put in the exact same code and set me free. I also spend far more time than I should stood in hurricane-force winds loading the system/calling the office to get the key code, entering it into the old fashioned key safe, to find the door is already unlocked.

I'm sure every community nurse has a special section of their brain reserved just for these 4-6 digit passwords so we can get to you with minimal delay (you try standing in the rain for ten minutes with all your kit waiting for care staff to let you in – gets you off to a great start). With regular patients and care homes, we're usually pretty good at knowing every single one. Sometimes we don't actually know them, we just know the pattern on the keypad our finger needs to make to get us through the door. I find it an impressive skill in itself to remember all these numbers, especially when it's been a busy week and I don't even know what day it is.

The Naivety of Students

I like students. I think this is because I was one not so long ago and remember how important it is as a trainee to have an approachable mentor to help you learn. It makes the world of difference when you don't feel like you're about to ask a stupid question and you end the day having learned something you started in the morning being absolutely clueless about. It can actually make or break students, having good mentors. I've always taken juniors under my wing for this reason, whether it's first years when I was in my final year, nursing students as a Band 5, or even supervising new start nurses in the community.

Some student nurses I've been massively impressed by. Their logical thinking, their patient interaction, their aspirations. I love to see eager students who are keen to learn and develop. Others, I have wondered how they even got through their interview. I've had a student who spent so much time on her phone on a shift with me, she's lucky she didn't get thrown out of the car at the next set of traffic lights. I've heard about a student telling a very experienced senior colleague, "there's nothing you can teach me". I'm sorry but if a student said that to me, even now in my own nurse infancy let alone after however many decades of experience, professionalism might go out of the window for a few moments, quickly followed by the student. A reputation for disrespect is certainly not what you need in life, especially not when trying to pass nursing training, but to be honest, speaking to senior staff like that, I think one would seriously need to reconsider their career path all together.

Middle students are the cutest. They're starting to recognise the types of skills you need as a nurse, but are not quite confident enough in themselves to act on them. They try, and I would never ridicule them for that. No question or suggestion is stupid, but I have had some secret giggles to myself. I had an end-of-first year student with me once, quite shy but I think she was like me when I was learning – quiet while I figured things out. We were visiting a regular diabetic one day, a man just four years away from seeing one century old, and we found him in the kitchen, trying to pick up a crate of bitter off the floor. I could see it now; he would fall, crack his head open, and then we've opened a whole new can of worms. So I told him to let me get it, picked it up (demonstrating flawless moving and handling skills of course, for the benefit of my impressionable student) and put it on the kitchen side. When we got back to the car, my sweet little student was ever so worried about him. "Is he an alcoholic? Do we need to refer to substance misuse?"

Heck child calm down!!

This guy was 96. I'm certainly not shipping him off to spend his final days at Alcoholic Anonymous. Aside from the quite high possibility that, given his choice of language most days, he'd probably be banned within the month, I explained why I wasn't concerned. Yes, he did have rather a lot of alcohol in that cupboard, but at 96, I very much doubt we would get very far asking him to reconsider his lifestyle choices. His blood sugars were stable (high but stable), he didn't stink of booze, and never have I seen him so under the influence that I was concerned for his safety (apart from trying to pick up a pack of eight cans off the floor, using his Zimmer frame for balance). And for some reason, I would rather see ten unopened bottles of wine in someone's house, than ten empty wine bottles (we've all had those 'last minute didn't know what to get' birthday/Christmas presents).

As a student, we're taught to read between the lines, but not to make up issues that aren't there to begin with. Her level of concern was nice, it was the first time she'd met him (we've seen him daily for years for insulin) so she didn't know, but my goodness she needs to snap out of the habit of making unnecessary work for herself. On a serious note, however unnecessarily over the top her reaction was, it's a prime example of how we holistically assess every patient we see, at every opportunity.

You Should Have Been Here Yesterday

So should you.

You Should Have Been Here Yesterday Pt 2

Unlike practice nursing, district nursing works more on a clinical need basis rather than appointment times. Our nurses only have so many hours in a day, so sometimes where more urgent clinical situations have arisen during the day – the SOS calls – we need to prioritise these and it may lead to patient visits getting deferred to the next day. We do our best to make sure this doesn't happen but we can't magic staff out of nowhere. Most of the time, patients are understanding of this, and even though we don't want them to feel as though they're not important to us, we don't argue with them when they say, "some people need you more than me".

Other patients are less understanding. Don't ask me why but it's in these instances, you really learn to keep your mouth shut. Only in our heads do we say, "I'm sorry, next time someone is in agony whilst they're dying, I'll explain that their pain relief will have to wait because I've got to come and redress your leg because you've taken the bandaging off **again**." Only in our heads do we say "I'll leave that blocked catheter, he can't need to pee that bad, the pipe is just for show". We let them have their rant, put on a smile and apologise (we do mean it) but after we've ended the courtesy call to let them know what's going on, it's forgotten. Honestly. Our priority is with the SOS we've just deferred the visit for. We've rebooked the patient in for a 'do not defer' visit tomorrow, what more can we do?

When we get to such patients' houses and are met immediately with "you were supposed to be here yesterday" (not hi how are you or anything), our level of compassion can dip ever so slightly for a moment. Just don't even start. "Yes, Mr C we were supposed to come yesterday but as we explained on the phone **yesterday**, we had to attend an emergency call out". The worst bit about this is when you don't know whether the patient is genuinely being rude or is just having you on. Either way, not funny, don't bother.

If It's Funny, I'll Laugh

"Are you allergic to anything?"
    "Only needles…"

"Do you have any hearing difficulties?"
        "What?"

"Can I do this…?"
            "What if I said no?"

Some patients bless them, try to be funny. The first time you hear it, yes it's funny, well done. The second time, I'll laugh but partly because I'm not sure if you remember that you've already told me. The third time I will finish the question for you. Past four, just be quiet. Again, another example of things I've heard so many times, if I were paid a pound for every time, I might be able to start saying I am in this job for the money.

The consent joke in particular is quite annoying. If I ask you if I can give you an injection/redress your wound/take a photograph, and you're think you're being funny by saying no, I won't take that as a joke. I will take it as a refusal of consent, something that's a big deal in nursing. If you say no, I won't do it, because if I did, legally it could be construed as assault. Even if we've heard that joke a hundred times from you, there is no room for complacency because that one time you say no, might be the one time you really mean it.

138

The hearing difficulties joke is a favourite with male patients over the age of 60. When I first started doing assessments alone (without supervision of another nurse while I settled in – the famed supernumerary period), I fell for that joke more times in one sitting than I have fingers to count on. One patient had me repeat the question four times in a row, the little bugger. I am becoming wise to this now and unless I have a reason to believe otherwise (i.e. obvious presence of a hearing aid – this is getting more difficult to see now with new technology) you get a two-shot lee-way. After that, I will politely suggest any more what's and you'll be a lightbulb.

Other jokes go so over my head, I wonder if they're not actually jokes and I'm treating a racist, a homophobe, or a chauvinist, none of which I have time for and will not entertain by participating in the conversation. Healthcare professionals have a tendency to develop a dark, sometimes twisted, sense of humour in their jobs, and it's used as a coping mechanism for the daily stresses and pressures. The saying 'if we didn't laugh, we'd cry', has never been more true than when working in healthcare. It doesn't make us bad people, as long as we keep it out of earshot of patients and never compromise professionalism because of it. Most of the time we don't even mean it…

Behind Every Nurse

A nurse would struggle without a good team. You know my views on carers referring to themselves as 'just a carer'. I've been a support worker and on some occasions, I've been the one to get nurses and doctors out of sticky situations. Now, as the Band 5 myself, I would be nowhere without my healthcares. Absolutely worth their weight in gold. I will maintain that for the rest of my career, that behind every good nurse is a great healthcare.

I've picked up on a potential medication error in a critical care environment, written by a new junior doctor (as in not far from the first Wednesday in August new) – they had prescribed far too high a dose of a blood thinner given the condition and history of the patient. I may have only noticed this because I was also a trainee nurse, but that shift I was working as clinical support and so my suggestion that the dosage was revised went down like a lead balloon. Very much a 'what do you know, you're just a healthcare' attitude and clear annoyance that I had picked this up, but essentially it saved the patient from a potentially catastrophic bleed. I can deal with the bad feelings knowing that deep down, I'm pretty sure the new doctor was thankful that I had mentioned it quietly on the side (although at the time, they made me feel so small, part of me felt like standing in the middle of the ward and announcing it quite publicly).

When I hear other people refer to carers in derogatory terms as 'just a carer' or 'only a band 2', I can almost feel the internal rage boiling over. I will acknowledge when I believe that some tasks are out of the scope of practice for support workers, and here I might say 'not trained', but in terms of advice and knowledge junior staff can offer, never underestimate it. I 'outrank' my healthcare by two pay bands and a degree but he outshines me by 25 years of NHS experience. He is one of the first people I will go to for advice, and I never dismiss any information he has to offer. Although I'm technically his senior, I'd never carry around the attitude that I am, something I've seen far too much. I also feel like this towards my ambulance crew colleague – ECAs are a band 3 but he would have wiped the floor with me in an emergency situation. And a driving test. Think of the banding system like a building; it can go 5, 6, 7 stories high, but without sturdy foundations, the whole lot will collapse.

Never look down on your housekeepers either – if they decide you deserve to clean your own mess up, guess what you'll be doing. Never look down on support workers, they will have your back more times than you'll realise. Just as doctors 'shouldn't' look down on the nurses, because we save their behinds every single working day.

I Can't Get to the Practice Nurse

I love it when patients inadvertently drop themselves in it. As per criteria, if they can get to the surgery, off to the surgery they go, so we can see patients who are actually stuck in their homes. It's so frustrating when we're driving along to our visits, and see our patients walking down the street. Especially when at their next visit (which is when we're all raring to go to discharge them to the PN) they deny being able to go out at all. Professionally, we can't stand there and say they're lying; there's no proof and it wouldn't do our patient care reports any good.

Sadly, it's not our problem if you might have to get a taxi/bus/heaven forbid walk, to the surgery. There are some exceptions where we know patients can get out and we keep them on the caseload – it all depends what they're on the caseload for. We're not harsh on purpose, we simply don't have the time or capacity for visits when the patient is capable of going to the surgery.

Sometimes patients slip up and it really makes our day. We don't like people abusing the service because it's easier for us to go to them. They're the minority of course, but they do exist. I've come across patients who request specific times or who aren't in when I visit because they're at the shop/pub a little bit further away than their surgery (but then insist that they're restricted to the confines of their back garden at the very furthest). I've come across patients who can't leave the house without their husband/wife (who it turns out only works three half-days a week and takes said patient along to pick the kids up from school) – it's amazing what a bit of 'pointless chit-chat' can reveal. Playing this game with us instantly puts you on our hit list and we will make it our mission to discharge you at some point in the very near future, even if it means sending in some of the 'harder' nurses (my team have a select few who will go in and get them gone, no messing about). That's if you don't discharge yourself of course.

At a recent first visit (NP = new patient), after a conversation about how their mobility is so poor they can't possibly get to the practice (and me falling for it), I kept the patient on the caseload for wound care for twice weekly reviews. Unfortunately, I couldn't make the second visit due to unforeseen circumstances, so I rang them to apologise and promise I would get to them the next day. Patient was happy with this, I engaged in a bit of 'pointless chit-chat', asked how the wound was and how they've been etc. No problems reported. Apparently, the wound was feeling so good, the patient proceeded to tell me, "you'll be really impressed I think, I bet you could send me to the surgery after seeing it tomorrow".

Simple fact you've just said that to me means that's exactly what I'm going to do. Bright spark.

It's a Miracle

Following on from reduced mobility meaning patients can't get to the practice nurse, I can remember being on a community placement in my first year. We were visiting a patient with a pressure ulcer on his sacrum because he couldn't walk at all and so spent his days in bed. The wife was quite anxious and was one of those (annoying) relatives that hovers over your shoulder and tells you to do it this way and that way, how to do your job basically. Thinking back now, I never noticed any moving and handling equipment like a hoist, in the house. This guy's wound wasn't healing because apparently the dressing kept 'falling off' (his wife was taking it off daily to give the wound a good 'clean') and because he was bedbound.

Imagine our faces when we opened the front door to see him hot-footing it across the landing back to his bedroom…

SOS My Legs Are Wet

One of the top three SOS calls is 'leaking legs'. This means the legs are leaking fluid/wound exudate and it has come through the dressings (strikethrough). If there is wound fluid coming through to the outside of the dressing, the dressing choice/frequency needs to be reassessed; it could indicate deterioration or infection. In hot weather, wet dressings could attract flies which will get a bit romantic on the dressings, leaving lots of eggs, and you know what fly eggs turn into.

Of course, without seeing them, we can only take the caller's word for it. Some patients know this and, as with the ambulance service, know all the right things to say to put them at the top of the list. Some patients are a little bit overcautious. Some patients are confused and think their legs are leaking when in fact, they've urinated all over themselves (which to be fair, is still a condition we don't want you sitting in, for your own sake as well as your wound).

We have a 24-hour window for responding to SOS leaky legs but generally, being an SOS, we aim for a same day visit. The nurse may postpone one visit to attend this call, only to find there is no leaking leg at all. These calls usually come from elderly people with cognitive issues so we can't really get mad with them. Of course, we're frustrated inside but for all we know, it could have been like they'd stepped in a puddle or they could have been absolutely p**s wet through with blood. Until we get there, we never truly know.

I attended an SOS call for bilateral leaking legs today, called in from a care home. What a waste of time. Well, kind of. They weren't leaking – the outer dressings were slightly damp but the fluffy bandaging underneath (used to shape the leg) and the actual absorbent dressing was bone dry. What's more likely is that the patient had spilled a cup of tea or something. However, the visit wasn't a total waste of time, because this patient was always wandering about and the bandaging had slipped slightly. When this happens, it becomes a falls risk if it comes undone and there's the potential for it to start rolling, forming a kind of rope – rope around the legs isn't great for pressure damage. So I changed the dressings, amended future visits (he won't need a visit tomorrow now) and suggested to the carers when an SOS should be called through. Luckily, today was 'reasonably quiet' and I had space to fit him in. If I had cancelled a visit to attend, I may have been a little less polite.

Some patients call in 'leaky legs' in the late afternoon but we are so busy, we refer to the evening service. Who are then turned away because the patient is in bed or it's too late or whatever other reason. Please, if you're going to call in as an urgent request, please don't be picky about when we get to see you. Sadly, if we don't attend immediately, some patients also call the ambulance service. Vicious circle.

Where's My F**king Dog?!

Out on my rounds today, on the rural routes, I came across a car that had very recently flipped over onto its roof. There was a young man (teenager – probably just passed his test and took the corner too quick) waving me past. Hmmm, that wouldn't do my conscience any good now would it. "Is anybody injured?" I asked him as I pulled up alongside the now upside-down Peugeot. "No, nobody's injured, everyone's out, just a bit of a shock love" he replied. Bit of a shock? Understatement? I was a 'bit shocked' and I only saw the car, I wasn't in it. He must have been doing some speed to completely flip the car over.

I was on my way to an essential visit, he didn't appear injured and his friends had just pulled up in a Transit van and were grimacing at the state of the car. As I was driving off, I heard the van driver shouting "where's my dog, where's my f**king dog?!" I was worried now – where was the dog? I handle animal harm a lot less well than people harm strangely enough, and wondered whether his dog was okay for the next hour. But in that situation, with young men so irate and potentially aggressive, I didn't feel comfortable stopping and helping any further – it was a rural road and there were three men (and a transit van), one of which was absolutely fuming that he couldn't find his dog. I am a woman on my own, my uniform encourages respect but it's not magic. Had there been human injury, of course I would have helped, but there wasn't so I would have been a bit stupid to put myself at risk in the midst of this for the sake of a dog that had ran off. The three men could look for it.

I did drive past on my way home just to make sure everything was alright, and the car had been removed.

Whatever You Say Ma'am

Given that the majority of our patients are over 70, it's no surprise that a fair few of them have served in the Forces in their younger years. With some patients, this really shows in their authoritarian personalities and how particular they are with dressings. I've been told that I'm not putting the bandages on right and I should be scrubbing the floors with a toothbrush until I learn how to do it properly (this came in as an SOS the next day because he'd taken them off). I've had comments regarding how immaculately 'pressed' my uniform is, am I going on parade? I've even been told to stand up straight (never mind I've just been bent over in an almost foetal position for the last half an hour bandaging your lower legs). What's common with all of these patients though, is the respect they have for medics and their uniforms.

I spent time with the practice nurse at a Royal Air Force base during my training and I loved to see the Officers walking around in their uniforms, so perfectly laundered and with a posture that would put the Stickman to shame. I enjoyed watching the hustle and bustle of base life, watching the uniforms running to and fro across the runway and queuing for their routine medical. It's a nice feeling knowing that the respect I have for Forces personnel is reciprocated.

One gentleman in particular stands out to me because he insisted on calling me 'Ma'am' throughout the entire visit, at every visit. Yes, Ma'am, no Ma'am (three bags full Ma'am). It was quite a strange feeling really, being referred to as Ma'am all the time when I'm young enough to be his granddaughter (did I mention he called me Ma'am?). It was very clear how much gratitude he had for medical personnel and that the Forces were still very much at the forefront of his mind. Being called Ma'am so much, I think I did stand up quite straight during his visits.

This same gentleman also gave me a right telling off at a later date, because I apparently told him previously that I had two children (when again, the last time I looked, no I didn't). Again, reminding me that because two nurses on the same team both have brown hair, we must be the same person. Can you imagine if I'd have told him I wasn't married either?!

Turning of the Tables

I knew I recognised the name. New patient on the caseload – my secondary school Science teacher. Wow.

After my first visit, I left feeling incredibly humbled. My my, how the tables had turned. Someone who had played a massive part in the education that equipped me to develop a career in nursing, now needed my help to heal. I still felt the need to call them by their 'teacher name', even though I was the 'authority figure' now. Small world. I found it very moving to support them during their time of need, especially after they had personally supported me during my GCSEs and A-Levels, the passing of which allowed me to be where I am today.

What was even more moving, was that even after 15 years, they recognised my name on my name badge and remembered me for being a perfectionist and commenting on their less than perfect spelling. I thought I kept my head down at school, never really stood out, but I guess I didn't do a good enough job because recently another of my teachers came to be under my care. I don't say anything at the time, to avoid any potential embarrassment on their part, but just as we parted ways, he asked "Did I teach you?" Sixteen years and however many pupils later, it's quite nice really that my old teachers remember me, and I promise it's not because I was a hell-raising demon child at school.

Building Up Rapport

The patients we see are at a very vulnerable point in their lives. Many faces come and go every day, people who were once independent and active, now struggle with everyday things, the families of people who are nearing the end of their lives feel passed from pillar to post.

It's hugely important to build a good working relationship with patients and their families, especially in tense environments such as palliative support. Some patients ideally need to have the same 2-3 people visiting, in order to provide continuity of care. Personally, I like to see the same person regularly throughout their episode of care, because I can become well-read in terms of their needs and history. This is obviously not always practical and most patients adapt fairly well. Some however, don't react well to different faces every day and understandably so. Some patients can see three different pairs of carers a day, plus a different nurse; it's no wonder people can begin to feel overwhelmed having so many people coming and going in and out of their home all the time. Here, we try and send in the same staff members where we can.

Building a good rapport with patients isn't just something that is important to community nursing, but to the healthcare profession in general. Many times, I've seen patients who haven't mentioned their concerns to the care staff who are there 24/7, instead waiting until a member of the DNT visit; one patient didn't report chest pain for two days because he was waiting for one of the DNT team whom he trusted the most. That person was me. Being especially fond of this patient, I freaked out a little bit to myself; he'd waited two days for me, what if I was on annual leave?! That in itself, shows how important it is to build trust and approachability with patients. Luckily he was okay but he could have been having a heart attack.

Some people are hard to break and it can take many visits before they finally 'let you in'. When they do though, it's completely worth it. The thank you cards and the boxes of chocolates in between the verbal abuse remind you how fulfilling and rewarding this job is, and how you're making a difference to someone's life. Sometimes, it's more subtle; you gradually see the patient relax and notice little things that hint they are feeling more relaxed with you. I visited a very quiet, very reserved man who was on the caseload for daily bilateral legs. Never very chatty, to the point where it sometimes made me feel uncomfortable because I wasn't sure how to break through that barrier. After seeing him 4-5 times, he started talking to me about the football season. Now, football is something I know less than nothing about but this was a possible way in, so I asked who was playing (the match was between don't know and not sure), who did he place his bets on, what else is he interested in. I was hoping to find some common ground. His other interest was cricket. Again, something I'm clueless about (all sport in general to be honest).

Every time I visited, he would mute the TV. In one way I didn't mind because it allowed me to hear the winces of pain under his breath that he tried to hide when I cleansed the half a centimetre-deep ulcers encircling his legs, but in another way, as we had nothing to talk about (being daily visits, I'm sure he was fed up of being asked if he was eating and drinking okay), the silence could be quite unsettling. I repeatedly told him he didn't have to turn the sound off, but he was insistent.

On my perhaps seventh visit, he asked me if I could move a chair for him. YES! I absolutely can do that for you. The next day, we spoke about the goldfinches in the garden – he'd not seen them for a while. Today, he muted the TV, saw it was me visiting, and unmuted it. To me, that's a massive breakthrough. He even asked if the fan was bothering me. We had a little chat about whether he preferred morning or afternoon visits, and I left feeling like we'd made progress in that sometimes tricky area that is the patient/practitioner relationship. He's comfortable enough with me to just let me get on with things, and I think it took his mind off the pain slightly as well.

More Teas, More Wees

Being on the road poses its own problems in terms of bathroom opportunities (for us ladies anyway – I'm sure our male HCA doesn't have an issue). I tend not to drink a lot out on the road, coincidentally especially in the summer, when I'm actively trying to make sure I'm drinking enough. Between long visits and houses you really don't want to even set foot in let alone ask if you can use the bathroom, the bladder can become subject to quite a bit of abuse. On busy days, it's not unusual to have the first wee before leaving home, the second at lunchtime and the third when the work day is done. We are the biggest hypocrites ever regarding urination. When I was on placement on the day surgery ward, one of the key questions we asked when deciding if someone was ready for home was "have you passed urine?" If you hadn't, you're not leaving until you do (general anaesthetic can wreak havoc on the body and cause urine retention). We encourage patients to drink enough to keep the urine straw-coloured and yet we are the worst culprits for a) not drinking enough and b) not going when we need to.

Many patients ask if I'd like a cup of tea. Yes, I would absolutely bloody love a cup of tea! But, aside from not having the time, my motto has become 'more teas, more wees'. If I accepted every cup of tea offered throughout the day, I would have to cut my workload in half just to accommodate the cuppas and toilet breaks.

I personally don't like to ask patients if I might use their bathroom but once the water's running when I'm washing my hands, I start to think I could be a poster child for pelvic floor exercises.

Names Not Numbers

PLEASE if you must give your house a name, don't get rid of the number all together. I've noticed this especially in little villages, everybody has a sodding name for their house and no number. I've driven up and down streets several times before finding Wisteria Cottage and Orchard House (neither of which has wisteria or fruit trees to give it away). Chapel House is nowhere near the church, White Gables is so overgrown with ivy I haven't a clue what colour the house is, and as for other weird and wonderful names like Lynn Dene and other versions of names/places, don't even get me started.

While we're at it, if you must name your house, please ensure that the one and only sign saying so, isn't obscured by plants or cars, or only readable in broad daylight on one side of the road only.

Christmas Day on Christmas Eve

Community nursing is a 24 hours a day, 365 days a year service. We work weekends, bank holidays, Easter Sunday and Christmas Day. In my first year of qualification, I offered to work Christmas Day – partly because I believed that I would cop for it anyway, having joined the team halfway through the annual leave year when requests and holidays had already been dished out, and NQNs get s**t shifts, and partly because my mentoring nurse advised me to.

To keep things fair, we have to work a certain number of public holidays per year, and in the community, the general 'rule' is that you work at least two of the five Christmas period 'hot-days' (Christmas Eve, Christmas Day, Boxing Day, New Year's Eve and New Year's Day). I was unofficially advised that patients tend to be too busy with family and friends on Christmas Day and don't really want the nurse coming so it's generally a light shift.

That nurse wasn't lying. Christmas Day was one of the most blissful shifts I've ever worked. I had my Christmas Day (and associated festivities – dinner, presents etc.) with my family on Christmas Eve so I didn't really miss out, and on Christmas Day the only visits required on the most part, were insulins. I had the majority of my calls finished by 11am and spent the afternoon on-call before my evening insulin visits. I was available for SOS calls, which didn't come through, so I was able to catch up on travel expenses, spend more time than normally allowed with

158

patients, and generally have a lovely relaxed day. Which is probably the only time I will ever say that about a nursing shift.

You Do This I'll Do That

Teamwork. Important in any job. Even if you were stranded on a desert island alone, you would work with the sun and the tides to optimise your chances of survival (except me, I would probably die from dehydration simply from crying and be found face down in the sand). As said before, the NHS is like a big work family and when it's broken down into its smaller department/units/teams, that bond is greatly enhanced. Sometimes in the DNT, planned visits are reallocated during the day to allow for skill mix, SOS calls and traffic issues.

In most cases, the way the team work together to ensure efficient service is something that continues to amaze me. Even in instances where I've overlooked it or not realised, it's been brought to my attention by a phone call from a colleague to say "I'm next door, do you want me to see Mr S while I'm here?" Sometimes the clinical need or skill required means a visit swap isn't possible, but where it is, it allows us to be more efficient with our time and reduce the possibility of visits being delayed. Looking out for your colleagues is one of the strengths of the NHS team.

Being a community nurse can be somewhat isolating sometimes – on a busy day or a clinic day, the only time you may come into contact with another member of staff is at handover, and that's if visits and traffic allow. Maintaining communication is essential not just for the job in hand, but for personal sanity. And where colleagues don't keep you sane, they keep you company in insanity.

Documentation is Everything

Mental capacity is a complicated issue but the basic principle is, every individual has capacity to make a decision unless it's been proven otherwise. It only applies to single decisions – just because someone doesn't have capacity to decide whether they're safer in a residential home (and who would want to leave their lifelong home), it doesn't mean they don't have capacity to make every other decision in their life (including personal care), and even if the decision isn't one we would necessarily think is right for them, it's doesn't mean they don't have capacity to make it. Mental capacity is really important when patients give consent.

If someone refuses an injection, as long as they can make an informed decision to reject it, that is their right.

If someone declines personal care (even if they're living in far from hygienic conditions), if they have capacity to make that informed decision, and this includes being able to weigh up the pro's and cons of living in squalor, that is their choice. It's a difficult concept for me to grasp because I have a habit of practically completely bleaching my entire house every Friday night. A basket full of ironing to me is a disaster.

For us as a community team, it's a difficult area. Generally, most of the time, patients don't refuse nursing care. Other times, they refuse all input from the DNT. If they have capacity, there is absolutely nothing we can do about it. If someone has capacity and chooses to live in unsanitary conditions knowing it will cause/prolong illness, we have to respect that. Even if we leave the house scratching our ankles and feeling like we need to shower immediately. If someone refuses an injection, we have to respect that. Sometimes people joke "what if I said no". Then no it is, I can't do it, simple as. I'm not going to beg you. We can act in the best interests of a patient but we won't physically restrain patients to provide treatment. It puts them at risk of harm, and us. We will seek assistance from the mental health team.

What puzzles me though, is how some people don't have capacity but can sail through mental capacity tests. Alarm bells would be ringing in my head immediately if someone passed an assessment but still insisted they could cure leg ulcers by spitting on them (yes this is true and has happened). The test on one day might declare capacity present, but on our next visit, it might be a bad day.

It follows the principles of the Mental Capacity Act – picking the best time of day etc. – to enable full interaction, but some situations actually scare me and on bad days, I really wish I could carry around a mental health professional in my pocket. There's a fine line between lacking capacity, non-compliance, and pure mental illness; the difficulty lies in proving which one it is. This is where the importance of documentation is highlighted. Aside from being a legal requirement, accurate documentation can be the difference between consent and assault. Where memory/capacity fluctuates, consent may have been gained at the time of the visit, but later on it may be reported that the patient didn't want the intervention or give permission.

It's important to cover our own backs in what can sometimes feel like' defensive practice'. Even members of the public and care staff can mishear things, misconstrue information, and we've had many incidents where a patient or staff member has told one of our team "so and so said this" when actually we didn't. This is why it's so important to accurately record any action, or reason for lack of action, whether it's physical contact or a telephone call, in a timely manner, working to the rule 'explain it to the coroner'. A colleague was recently selected to give evidence at a coroner's court for an unexpected, potentially suspicious death, but because their documentation was spot-on, they didn't need to attend in the end. The Courts had everything they needed. If it wasn't written down, it didn't happen.

Is There Anyone Else While I'm Here?

Care homes make up at least a third of our caseload. To reduce travelling time and keep our team running efficiently, it isn't unusual for a staff member to see four or five patients on the same day, in the same care home. If time allows, we will often ask the care staff if there's anyone else that needs seeing 'while we're here'. We are offering the opportunity for you to work with us. So, if we ask if there's anyone else, and you say no, please make sure you mean it. Don't call through an SOS for a 'red bottom' two hours later for something that could have been mentioned whilst we are in the care home, because now all of our team are miles away with other visits. Unfortunately, unless it's a visit that falls into the 'four-hour window', we won't be able to get out to you again today. You had your chance.

How Much Do I Owe You?

One thing that never ceases to make me smile in this job, is when I've seen an elderly patient, usually with dementia, after I've completed whatever I'm there for, asking "How much do I owe you?" Perhaps it's a generational thing, quite possible when the patient was born before the birth of the NHS in 1948. It makes me smile, and in a strange way, makes me smile even more when the patient is so grateful when I remind them they don't have to pay me anything. It also reminds me how lucky we are as a nation to receive free healthcare. Okay, there will always be some that remind you that they 'pay their dues' but generally, when medical insurance is something that most other countries require before you even set foot in an office to see a medical professional, we are extremely lucky.

There are concerns with the privatisation of healthcare and reductions in the services provided, which are quite apparent in the media and talk amongst younger patients, but for now at least, most of the services provided by the NHS are free at the point of care. If you need life-saving surgery, you will have it. We don't need your bank details beforehand. I will politely remind people of this when people complain about waiting times and the cost of a prescription (and other such issues that, quite frankly, aren't under the control of a band 5 community nurse). Yes, we pay for prescriptions and dental treatment, but it's a small price to pay for managing what could otherwise be a much more serious condition. Those with certain long-term conditions are entitled to free prescriptions, contraception is free, all of the resources we use as a DN team are free to the patient. There is no bottomless pit of money and I dread to think of the state some people would be in if they couldn't afford to pay for medical care. Some patients on my caseload require specialised daily dressings – this could cost hundreds of pounds per month for an indefinite amount of time. This is why it's so important to use resources effectively and mindfully.

In a worst case scenario, if ten people who were living below the poverty line and who didn't have medical insurance, all required leg dressings each month that they couldn't afford, what would the alternative be? Sepsis? Death? Amputation? That's ten people needing an amputation they can't afford, with antibiotics they can't afford, all because they needed dressings they couldn't afford. An extreme example yes, and I'm aware that some treatments do cost the patient personally, but on the whole, what a fantastically lucky nation we are to have medical attention at our fingertips. Another reason I feel so strongly about the misuse of emergency ambulances – I'm running out of fingers to count the amount of times an ambulance has been called/deceived/manipulated into a free lift closer to home because someone couldn't afford a bus ticket....

Oh No It's You Again

"Oh no she's seen me. Busted". A highlight of my time as an NQN, chasing an 87-year old down the corridor in a care home when it's time for his insulin. Made my day.

Another 'care home insulin' also pulls the most delightful face at me when I visit in the evening for the second jab of the day. It tends to be mainly insulin patients that make these remarks and I can't blame them really. I wouldn't particularly like being stabbed and injected twice a day. I had the finger-prick blood spot test for iron levels at my most recent blood donation session and finger felt bruised for two days afterwards. I've seen fingertips almost blue from having to be pricked several times a day for years, they almost look like actual thimbles. Of course, none of the patients refuse the insulin but it does give me a giggle when they don't hide the fact that they're sick of seeing the blue uniform brandishing a needle at them.

My colleague doesn't get so much sweetness and giggles, having recently knocked on a patient's front door and being immediately asked "what the f**k do you want?" Charming.

More Photos for Facebook

We like photographs. It's easier to compare improvement and deterioration of a wound with photos and, especially with long-term wounds (the ones you've been seeing for precisely 4765 and a half days), it's easier to spot the difference if there is one. I always ask the patient if they'd like to see the wound (if they haven't or can't) because it gives them a better idea of what we're talking about, rather than us saying "yeah it looks good".

When we talk about a wound to each other we can say it has a yellow sloughy base with areas of over-granulation but the patient probably has no idea what we're on about (some do know, thanks to Dr Google). Some patients take the description as it's horrible and manky and the worst thing you've ever seen, while others don't realise how bad their wound actually is. Photographs show improvement and also pack a bit of punch when we need to explain why wounds aren't healing because the patient is taking the dressing off the moment we leave.

After a while, you get to know which patients you can have a joke with, and it causes a few laughs when you ask to take a picture of their bottom to update their profile picture. Of course, we remind them that it won't go on Facebook. We generally sell to the highest bidder and it's up to them where it goes.

Dealing with Threatening Patients

Bravest thing any man has ever said to me – "you realise I could snap your arm right now?" Considering I was there for a recatheterisation and it was said in front of a senior colleague, possibly not the brightest thing to say. I didn't feel threatened by the comment, I simply replied it was really impressive he decided to say that when I was about to shove a pipe down his penis and that I can use a little or as much anaesthetic gel as I please. My first time catheterising a male and that's the response I get when I was quite nervous anyway. I should have told him I'd never done it before and he was practice. My colleague was slightly more professional and advised that he would be reported to the police and charged with assault. Intended as a joke by the patient I'm sure, but my colleague's response demonstrated that 'jokes' like that aren't appropriate and wouldn't be tolerated.

Some patients are more intimidating than threatening, and in the situation above I might have been a little more unsettled had I been on my own. I documented it well (as technically it was a verbal threat) and didn't entertain the conversation any further than my senior's warning. In the community, I've never been in a situation where I've felt in danger or seriously threatened. There are areas that we aren't massive fans of visiting, and when there is risk to safety, we go in pairs. There's one particular patient who is quite sexually inappropriate verbally;

again we document everything. Although he's inappropriate with his comments, I've never felt endangered visiting him; it wouldn't be a problem taking out his kneecaps if I felt physically unsafe…

I seem to accept rude behaviour towards myself to a certain extent (perhaps ignore is a more suitable word?) but I will not tolerate my colleagues being spoken to with anything less than the respect they deserve. A&E staff wouldn't tolerate verbal or physical aggression (luckily physical aggression is rare in the community in my experience), so why should we, just because we're in a different environment. I should maybe look out for myself as much as I do my colleagues.

I have been physically hurt in the job, but never intentionally (to my knowledge anyway). I've been kicked in the stomach by patients with brain injuries, suffered crush fractures to my ribs by relatives flying through doors like a bull in a bloody china shop (this was impressive though – resulted in three weeks off sick and a further two weeks in light duties), and had the most awful teeth you can think of just centimetres from my bare arms.

My arms seem to be a hot spot for being verbally assaulted/threatened. During my training when I worked at the hospital, I was a one-to-one for a patient in intensive care one night, and it was the longest night shift in the entire history of long night shifts. I would have thought he 'should' have been too ill to practically pin me to the bed but he managed it. He was a 1:1 as he was a falls risk and basically, I spent thirteen hours making sure he didn't climb out of bed and take all the expensive ICU equipment with him. During the night, a nurse asked me to keep his arm still while she administered a medication through his cannula. I held his arm gently but firmly, and halfway through the drug admin, like lightning he grabbed me with his other hand, spun my arm around, and if I hadn't slammed myself into the side of the bed in a pose a contortionist would have been proud of, my elbow would have snapped like a twig. It was rather tender the next day. The strength of ill people never ceases to astonish me, where do they find it?

I've been pinched, punched, grabbed at, but unfortunately it's all part of the job. If any of it was intentional, believe me the police would be involved, but a lot of patients have cognitive issues, and it's these patients that pose the greatest 'risk'. Even my car has been victim to a hit and run in the line of duty, whilst I was inside a patient's house. That hurt me more than the bust ribs.

What is this Rash?

We are nurses. We are quite clever. But sometimes, we don't know everything. Sometimes we might know but you're best off seeing your GP for a confirmed diagnosis. Calling through an SOS because someone has had a rash for three days and asking if we can go and see what it is, I'm sorry but aside from not being commissioned to go out on diagnosis visits, we would probably advise you to contact the GP even **after** we'd seen it anyway, so we may as well cut out the middle man. Some patients and relatives feel they can approach us more than their doctor but we can't take on every job going.

One particular SOS call was a bit sensitive, because the patient and family seemed to have been passed from pillar to post and still didn't have any clear-cut answers. I readied myself to ring Mrs T, I wasn't expecting this call to be easy. Rash had been present for three days and she was really concerned. To be fair, she did sound worried over the phone but as I've said before, some people do unfortunately know how to act and say all the right things to get a visit. I advised that we couldn't diagnose over the phone and we can't send a member of staff out just to have a look because we don't provide that service (even if we did have spare staff at the time). I advised them to call the GP and then they would have prompt access to medicated cream or whatever treatment they might need. "But they won't come!" she cried. "Well they're bloody well going to have to, he's bedbound and he's their patient", and I'm ashamed to say it, I did say it as bluntly as that. The GPs not visiting their patients isn't our problem, we can't take on the extra work to make their lives easier. I've even had patients asking the GP is they can go to the surgery for an injection but they've been told no, the district nurses will come...

Really, this rash sounded like heat/sweat rash, but I hadn't seen it to say that with any conviction, and if they were really concerned about this three-day old rash, why hadn't they sought guidance sooner? In my experience, when people do this, it's never just a 'quick look'. It turns into this problem and that problem and a barrage of while you're here's.

NQN me in my first week would have probably sent someone (this is why they don't give triage to staff without that resilience – 'bitch-ability'). I have become a little bit harder in this job and I've had my eyes opened, both by getting to know the job and getting to know the patients. Triage is not a problem for me now. I don't mean that in a way that might put someone off community nursing, but any career that you throw yourself into will change you somehow, and I don't think it's changed me for the worst – being a pushover in nursing is not the way to get things done. You have to stand up for yourself as well as your patients – regarding myself, I admit this is a work in progress but I'm getting there!

When 'rashes' are brought up during a routine visit, things are a bit different. You can't really sit there with your eyes shut and your fingers in your ears singing "nope not looking at it". I was visiting a lady for rather nasty leg ulcers on both legs and she was a bit wobbly when I first arrived; with a tonne of bandaging hanging off her legs with painful ulcers, and quite probably spaced out on morphine, I wasn't overly concerned.

Whilst redressing her right leg, she showed me a 'rash' on her outer thigh – to me it looked like a bruise, and I still to this day haven't seen an image that matches what I saw (and of all the days I forget my camera and repeatedly see visions of it sat on my kitchen table). She wondered if it was a reaction to the antibiotics she'd been taking. The bruising was about the size of my outstretched hand, and looked like the purple bruising elderly people get when they're on blood thinners and they bang their arms. That fragile skin that instantly goes purple if you just look at it wrong.

Anyway, during general chit-chat (and you know I'm such a fan) she mentioned she'd not felt very well the day before and had had the shivers during the night, but she felt fine now. Red flag. At that time, I didn't make the link between the bruising on her thigh and the symptoms reported to me (very clearly new to the job – I'd know now 100%) but alarm bells were ringing. Linked to the bruising or not, I was concerned about the symptoms she'd reported. I asked her relative to call the GP for a visit and to call while I was there so I could talk to them if needed. I explained the situation and reported normal observations, and the doctor agreed to visit later that day.

Turns out, the doctor went to see the patient and admitted her to hospital for IV antibiotics for sepsis. The bruising was a septic rash, where the infection had overpowered the system and almost eroded the blood vessels in the skin, causing bleeding under the surface. I really struggled to explain the bruise to the team in handover, and I went over loads of images with the 'big boss' but none of them were the same as what I saw. I always double check I have my camera with me now.

Please Don't Touch

I can't pinpoint the **exact** cause of sepsis in the lady
with the leg ulcers; her observations were
unremarkable and she was usually doing housework
of some sort when we visited. She had just finished
antibiotics for an infection in a burn wound on her
leg, which was nowhere near the bruising, but
obviously they hadn't gained control of the infection,
and it had spread systemically.

Now, I don't want to point the finger as to where
the infection may have come from in the first place,
but during the visit when I asked the lady's relative to
call the GP, he offered to do the dressing while I
spoke to the doctor (he had been changing the
dressings between our visits if they were leaking
through). I asked if he had any gloves and he said no.
Enough said, stop talking. No, you ring the doctor, I
will finish this dressing. He must have been changing
the dressings 2-3 times per week (even though we
said this was too frequent – we would have visited
everyday if needed), and if he didn't wear gloves, it
doesn't take a genius to work out how infection might
have got in.

We don't mind you offering to change your own or
your relative's dressings; besides promoting self-
care, it takes a heck of a lot of work pressure off us,
and it works better for you in most cases as well. We
have someone on the caseload who takes care of her
partner's wounds every day (she's pretty spectacular
in what she does) with one visit a week from the DNT

to review. We will visit weekly – we won't leave you to fend for yourselves – but we will only agree to this if we're sure you can follow infection control procedures and provide care using an aseptic non-touch technique. Changing dressings on ulcerated legs without gloves, a) why would you even want to?! and b) **massive** risk of infection. Please don't touch.

I Hate to See You Go but Love to Watch You Leave

Elderly people can be so sweet. I have all the time in the world for them. They're full of lovely stories, little pieces of advice, gratitude. However, I do think sometimes they forget they're not actually 29 anymore.

A regular insulin patient, lovely guy, always full of beans, a patient I really enjoy seeing, one particular day decided to tell me after I had administered his insulin, "I hate to see you go" and as I walked off, followed it with "I like to watch you leave". I have no idea where he got that from but I walked out of that care home trying to make sense of what the hell I'd just heard. I'm not sure if I was a bit disturbed or just wanted to wet myself laughing.

Aim in life – to marry someone who will still say that to me when I'm 89.

Leaving Nursing for Aldi?

I read about it every day; hundreds of nurses are leaving the profession. It's sad that things have become so dire in terms of stress and low pay for the hours worked, that experienced nurses are leaving the profession completely. I've heard so many times in the media that managers at budget supermarkets get paid almost twice as much as registered nursing staff, and nurses are resorting to food banks to feed their families. I'm not saying being a supermarket manager isn't hard work, but given the nature of our jobs, the unpaid overtime, the devastating effect it can have on your sleep pattern/social life/family time, it's no wonder that nurses are becoming so frustrated they're leaving all together.

With so many nurses leaving to retirement, and fewer applicants to nursing degree courses, the last thing the health service needs is more staff leaving due to discontentment. A friend works for a rail company, directing trains in and out of the station, announcing it on the tannoy (a bit like the Fat Controller in Thomas the Tank Engine) – paid nearly ten grand a year more than me. With facts like this floating about, it's very clear that nurses aren't in the profession for the money, but I agree with the majority of the general public that we should be financially 'thanked' for what we do. The most integral people to society seem to get paid below what they deserve.

I think the worst thing to happen in recent years is to remove the training bursary. An academic colleague at the University I trained at has told me there has been a dramatic drop in applications since the nursing bursary was stopped. I'm not surprised in the slightest. I couldn't have done the training without it, and I still had to work two jobs alongside. The majority of nursing students are 'mature', which means they have mortgages and children and absolutely no chance of working extra hours on top of studying, to earn a living. The bursary acted like a wage for us, especially when we were on placement, but name one person who would work full time every week for less than £600 a month. Absolutely not. At top whack minimum wage, we should have been coming out with at least £1100. As nursing students, working full time as well as academic commitments and travelling, we were 'earning' £4 an hour.

Nursing students won't be willing to work full time, on top of study to be nearly 30 grand in debt by graduation just in tuition fees, let alone maintenance and support loans for living. People are nurses for the love of it, and they will struggle their hardest to get to where they want to be, but today's world is more practical – it's sad to see people give up on their dreams because they can't afford to chase them. It's also sad to see experienced nurses who are specialists in their fields, leaving because they can't cope with the stress anymore. I suspect things will change in a few years and the bursary will be reinstated, no doubt due to the 'shortage' of nurses (which we already have anyway).

Knowing the Value of Work-Life Balance

Being new in a nursing career, it's easy to want to seize the bull by the horns and go for every development opportunity you can get your hands on – probably a trait left over from being a student. It's admirable and everyone needs aspirations and goals. But it must not come at the expense of your personal well-being. Only today, I told our bank HCA (soon to go into her final year of nursing training), don't work through next summer, enjoy it.

During the first four or five months as an NQN, it was really easy to do extra work once I got home, told myself it's while I find my feet. Teamed with staff shortages, too many visits and not having little people or a husband to look after at home (in case my patients dare let me forget), pretty quickly I found myself working longer shifts to help out, doing 2-3 hours of overtime at home allocating work to staff for the next day, covering a whole team area alone during the day, and not really looking after myself as I should. Life became work, shower, eat, sleep. Rinse and repeat.

I'm quite tough and powered through for a good while, but when I hit the wall, my goodness did I hit the wall. I had used every last ounce of energy and became exhausted, not just physically but mentally. Not a good place to be when you have patients to look after, having nothing left to give. As an NQN I was taking on some of the responsibilities of a Band 6 and ended up trying to drive on an empty tank. Through the support from colleagues, friends and family, once I recognised what had happened, I said "no more". My poor healthcare has heard me crying down the phone more times than I had hot dinners in that period of time. I had some annual leave, refreshed and reverted back to my role as an NQN. Situations like this are why people go off sick with stress. That annual leave came at just the right time or that would have been me (I was reluctant to stay off work with fractured ribs let alone go off with stress).

I started heading down that road again a few months after (because I obviously didn't learn my lesson the first time round) but my HCA saw it coming and stopped me in my tracks before I hit yet another wall at full speed with the airbag turned off. I can't stress the importance of maintaining a healthy work-life balance, particularly when we're new to our careers. We want to impress, we want to grab every opportunity to better ourselves, but the fire needs fuel to burn. Support from colleagues is invaluable; they see what you see every day and know exactly where you're coming from, because chances are they've been through it too. Developing such a strong working relationship with my HCA (even though he's my 'junior', he's saved my marbles more times than I care to count – never think you're better than anyone) meant he was knocking down the walls almost as fast as I was heading towards them. When you're running on empty, mistakes are made, tempers are short, emotions are fragile. Everything becomes worse than it is and it's a heavy burden to take home to your loved ones.

In any profession, you must look after yourself. Go home, switch off. First rule (or is it the second?) I will teach a student; you are more than your job. Behave like it.

She Won't Bite

A lot of our caseload are residents in care homes and therefore usually have cognitive impairments. Some are pleasantly confused others can be aggressive. It's the aggressive personalities that unsettle me, because they're generally so unpredictable.

One lady in a care home who we visit twice daily for insulin, can be really cooperative in the morning, medication given with no issues. She often tells people "I love you, you bastard", with a big toothy grin. In the afternoon, it can be a whole different ball game. I don't even see her on my own anymore, I ask a member of staff to reassure her and act as a bit of a distraction for me. You don't really need arms waving around trying to hit you in the face when you have needles and blood sticks in your hands, and arms don't wave so much when they're giving someone a big snuggle.

She was being 'snuggled' one day, the carer was holding her hands and reassuring her, talking about her family visiting. The insulin needle went in and I had nearly finished the administration before she started trying to bite my arm. I don't want anybody biting me maliciously, let alone with oral hygiene like that (something the care home struggle to get compliance with), so even with the carer (nervously) laughing, "she won't bite you, she won't bite you", thank you but I will make that decision and I'm not willing to take the risk. I'm not taking someone else's word for it that I wasn't going to have mucky jaws clamped around my uncovered forearm, I've seen the scratch marks on staff members' arms and I don't fancy physical injury if I can help it.

Luckily, I finished the injection and she got the full dose of insulin but I ensure there's always a carer with me when I visit that lady (told you we needed you), and my colleagues are doing the same thing. Human bites are dirtier than animal bites, and I've no doubt hers would have been even dirtier. And knowing my luck, she would have been like a terrier and not let go until she'd shredded me to pieces.

Are You a Trainee?

Whether it's because of my youthful good looks (laugh out loud) or because patients just don't trust nurses like they do doctors, I've been asked on a few occasions, "are you a student?" Of life and nursing, I am continually learning yes. But on the other hand, being asked if I know what I'm doing is slightly patronising, because if I didn't I wouldn't be doing it. I have upset other healthcare staff before by refusing to do something that I wasn't competent to do, but I don't care. It's my registration at risk if I work outside of my capabilities, not theirs, so they can guilt-trip me all they like.

It does bring to light how substandard care can impact the patient's perceptions of healthcare professionals. This is mentioned quite often when I need to take blood from patients. I haven't missed a vein yet, but they don't know that. They only know they've had several unsuccessful attempts (without sounding disrespectful) by junior doctors. Junior doctors tend not to need to take bloods so much, as the nurses usually do it or there's a phlebotomist floating about, so when they do take blood it isn't always straightforward. Give them an artery to pierce and they're away, but veins seem to evade them. I reassure my patients with the same, what seems to be a pre-written script; if I can get blood from the agitated drunk swaying about on the bed singing football anthems in A&E, I can get yours. If I can get blood from the end of life patient whose veins have all but shut down and disappeared completely, I can get yours. And if I can get blood from those damn fake arms, I can get yours.

Aside from being a little annoying (and it is just a little), it's concerning how many patients seem to worry about being 'practised' on. No I'm not a student. I'm a qualified professional. Just because you haven't seen my face before it, it doesn't mean it's my first day. Please trust me. And please don't freak out at me if I do something slightly different to the way the last nurse did it; it doesn't mean I'm doing it wrong.

Last month I visited a patient to reapply compression bandaging to her leg ulcers. I was scrutinised more by her than any of my tutors during my management placement. I put the rubbish bag in the wrong place, I cut the stockinette **before** I washed her leg, and I set the required dressings out to my right instead of to my left. "That doesn't go on that side" – does it really matter? (I'm right-handed so to me yes it actually does matter but bigger picture here).
"The others don't open that first they open the others" – REALLY?!

I make sure I have everything ready before I start the task in hand. It's better for infection control and fluidity of the dressing change. I don't want to change my gloves every time I realise I've forgotten something – we get through enough pairs in one visit as it is (one visit I counted twelve glove changes, and yes they were all necessary). I want to know that everything is ready and waiting but my word, this seemed like a new thing to this lady.

"They usually get it out when they need it" and "they don't cut that until they've washed my leg". Who are **they**, who have inadvertently made my visit so bloody difficult?! I politely (and it was so sickly polite I surprised myself considering how frustrated she was making me) advised, it doesn't matter what order I do things in, as long as it's according to infection control, the end result is the same. "The others don't do it that way".

OH MY GOD!! My thought process went along the lines of, 'the others don't complain this much' along with practically chewing the inside of my mouth off to resist saying it out loud. Instead, what came out was, "we've all done the same training though" (said with a horrendously sweet smile on my face). That seemed to do the trick. She wasn't getting away with dictating to me which side I have the waste bag on and whether I put emollient on the gauze that I'm washing her leg with or in the water. I left that visit feeling a little bit drained. Seeing as we aren't allowed to tell the patient to bloody well do it themselves if they know best, it certainly hones your skills to have 'polite arguments'.

You've Discharged Them to Us, Let Us Decide

Referrals that come from hospitals: – unless it's come from a tissue viability specialist, we're unlikely to take your requests for daily visits for wound checks and to change an adhesive stickie over a surgical wound seriously. You've discharged them to us and referred them into our care. And if there's one thing community nurses are s**t hot at, it's wound care. So please, let us decide how often we see a patient. On a ward, there are nurses and HCAs present 24/7 to change dressings. We don't have that luxury.

We are unlikely to see the patient until clips/stitches need removing anyway so that's at least 7-10 days post-surgery (provided there's no complications) and we're not commissioned for wound checks – this is something the hospital should educate their patients about pre-discharge. If a wound needs daily visits (e.g. packing of a cavity after abscess drainage) we will assess it at the first visit, and then if it needs daily visits fine, but 9 times out of 10 it doesn't, and we will increase or decrease the frequency of visits as required. Requests from tissue viability teams, yes, we do take them a bit more as gospel, but otherwise leave it to us.

Without blowing our own trumpet, we know a lot more about leg ulcers and dressings than GPs and wound care is a particular gift that community nurses have. Telling patients that the district nurses will visit **every day** causes us a headache as we spend more time trying to explain that in fact they don't need us every day, than actually performing wound care.

Working Through Lunch and Overtime

We know we don't get paid for it but it's not an unknown thing for staff to work through their lunch break. I do it practically on a daily basis. There are always little jobs that you do in between your coffee and whatever gastronomical delight (meaning cheap sandwich from the local petrol station) you've chosen for lunch.

As a community nurse, my car is my office, I don't particularly want it to be my canteen as well, so some admin tasks I take to the office. Which usually means I'm doing it during lunch. I don't mind too much, because most of the day it's the only time I can sit at a proper desk and fill out order forms, do travel expenses and catch up on emails. Some days I can get a bit cross with myself (in hindsight of course) that I've worked through lunch yet again and promise myself I'm not doing it again. It lasts 24 hours.

At times, I've worked 2-3 hours of overtime at night when I get home, finishing off what I didn't get chance to do during the day that can't really wait (I won't get chance tomorrow either) or waiting for a call back from an out-of-hours doctors that I was expecting in the early afternoon. Due to the sheer quantity of visits, we rarely have time to complete incident reports or mandatory learning during the working day so they come home with us. As previously mentioned even on a good day when everything is on track, my computer system will decide it's not going to work properly to let me complete the last few bits of admin before home time. Naturally, when I arrive home it's my best friend again. if you're the type of person who will absolutely never in your life, do even one minute of overtime or work through your unpaid break on a relatively regular basis, a career in the NHS is not for you.

Complain, Please

Frustrated patients and their families often threaten to complain if they feel there's an aspect of their care they're not happy with. Some think it will scare us and as a result, we will do anything they ask. If you want to complain, please do. If you feel there's a problem, nothing will ever be done about it unless you raise a complaint. Don't use it as a threat thinking it will get you your own way. It won't. And while we're on the subject, don't slag our work colleagues off to us either. If you don't like them then please keep it to yourself because we're quite a close knit little work family, and some of us are very good friends out of work too.

Responding politely and handing out a complaints process leaflet soon sifts out those who have a genuine complaint and those who are just spitting their dummies out. A lot of the time, the patients are just frustrated that they're not improving and they want to blame someone (especially if non-compliance if the reason). It's usually frustration with the service as a whole, not just one person, but at times, and especially as a 'baby nurse', it can be quite difficult not to take it personally. You're the only one there, you're their sounding board.

Some patients are cognitively impaired and say they're reporting you, and you personally, for the most interesting of things. I've been threatened with a personal complaint because I refused to leave the clinical waste bag behind on the floor so the patient could show her daughter. No, I am not leaving a bag full of bloodied, stinking dressings behind, it's an infection control hazard and a falls risk. And it's gross.

"We'll see" she hissed at me with narrowed eyes. "We'll see about **you**".

Maggots

I have yet to come across this and I hope I never do as it might go on my list of things my stomach absolutely cannot tolerate, but colleagues have reported on several occasions, finding maggots in wounds. And I don't mean medical maggots that sort of live in a tea bag and are meant to be there. No, actual maggots. Larvae. Fly babies. It's been raised at least three times in the last three months, that staff have found maggots squirming around in either wounds or skin folds. I cringe just thinking about it. My professionalism might go to s**t if I ever discovered that.

Wet bandages are a key culprit – if the fluid can come out, stuff can go in and the staff member has been blissfully unaware until they remove the last layer of dressing and a load of maggots fall out. Recently, a co-worker reported that a patient's relative asked the nurse to check a sore foot, only to be confronted with maggots in the crevice underneath the toes. What happened to personal hygiene? On the plus side, maggots in the wound might do us a favour – they love eating dead and unhealthy tissue so all the wound beds would be nice and clean...

Just kidding. Medical maggots are specially bred and incinerated after use for infection control reasons.

Last Thoughts

Today was my last day as a Community Staff Nurse. It's not because I hate the job, even though some parts of this book come across like that. Maybe even most of it? There are two areas of healthcare I am passionate about – Emergency Care and Sexual Health, and it is this second specialism I'm moving into.

Finishing my working week on triage, I reflected on my first year post-registration during the half an hour drive home. I have learned so many skills in a relatively short space of time, and made friends for life. I've been involved in so many different cases, and I'm thankful that I am so healthy. I have gained more clinical skills to add to my portfolio, and (finally) discovered the type of nurse I want to be. Okay, Sexual Health has its stigma and isn't everyone's cup of tea, but I find the area absolutely fascinating and it allows me to be quite heavily involved in domestic violence and sexual assault safeguarding, two things I feel quite strongly about. I can take with me lots of knowledge learned from the community; the communication skills, the counselling skills, experience of safeguarding process, and a strong stomach.

On another positive note, I am now saying goodbye to overtime and weekend working, and the emotional tangles that I sometimes ended up in after dealing with end of life patients. Generally, most of my patients from now on, will walk into my clinic room,

and walk out again, with a consultation in the middle of it. I have more study coming up to pass a contraceptive health exam (told you nursing was a lifelong learning curve), and I will think of my colleagues on the road, braving the bad weather and freezing temperatures when I'm snug and cosy in a clinic room in the middle of winter hahahaha...
Some colleagues in particularly I will miss working with, but as you find when you work so closely with people, we will stay in touch and I've made two friends for life.

Would I recommend being a nurse to others? Yes, absolutely, but only if you have what it takes. You can't learn to be a nurse. Prospective students need to understand that to be a good nurse, effective communication is the single biggest skill you will use. Clinical skills can be taught but good interpersonal confidence can't be faked in my opinion. It needs an inherently compassionate nature, resilience, and strength.
I would also recommend community nursing. There are some horror stories flying about out there that newly qualified nurses shouldn't do this area and that area, that they should go for an 'easier' specialisms when they first start out. I was offered positions with Medical Emergency Assessment and Neonatal Intensive Care – I don't imagine that they would have been the easiest of positions for an NQN but if they didn't think NQN's could do it, they wouldn't have advertised for them.

I was also told that newly qualified nurses shouldn't work and aren't usually employed in the community due to its wide-ranging nature and need for certain 'personality skills'. Rubbish. The skills I have learned working with the District Nursing Team are the single biggest career benefit of working there as an NQN. As far as post-registration jobs go, I couldn't have picked a better area in terms of improving my skillset and self-confidence.

Now I've secured a job in Sexual Health, I'll be building my career here and in a few years, I want to undertake a Masters Degree in Advanced Clinical Practice. While I'm starting as a novice CaSH nurse, undertaking exams and role-specific training to equip me to do the job effectively, I'll be utilising the people skills I learned in the community. However, due to the nature of the specialism, I may not be writing a book titled 'Confessions of a Sexual Health Nurse'…

Glossary

A&E	Accident and Emergency. Also known as the ED (Emergency Department). Contrary to popular opinion, it does **not** mean Anything and Everything.
CaSH	Contraceptive and Sexual Health.
CCU	Coronary Care Unit – intensive care for poorly hearts, usually after a heart attack.
CPD	Continuing Professional Development – ongoing study to maintain skills and knowledge. Requirement for nurses to maintain their PIN and registration.
DN	District Nurse - Band 6 with a specialist qualification.
DNT	District Nursing Team.
DVT	Deep Vein Thrombosis – blood clot in the deep veins of the leg. Emergency.
ECA	Emergency Care Assistant – Band 3 member of an ambulance crew.
ECG	Electrocardiogram – results in that pretty and (hopefully) up and down picture of the heart impulses.
ED	Emergency Department. Also known as Accident and Emergency.
GP	General Practitioner – doctors at the surgery.
HCA	Healthcare Assistant – otherwise known as clinical support, NAs

	(nursing assistants) or support workers. Bands 2-3.
ICU/ITU	Intensive Care Unit/Intensive Treatment Unit.
IV	Intravenous – straight into the vein.
MDT	Multi-Disciplinary Team – all the professionals involved in a patient care pathway.
MEAU	Medical Emergency Assessment Unit – a ward you stay on for up to three days while they figure out what's wrong with you.
NHS	National Health Service – (Mostly) free healthcare system of the United Kingdom founded in 1948.
NP	New Patient – patient new to the DNT caseload.
NQN	Newly Qualified Nurse – what you are from first registration until you complete your preceptorship. Baby nurse.
OT	Occupational Therapist – specially trained therapists who help patients to increase their independence to do activities that matter to them e.g. provide shower rails to enable patients to continue to wash independently.
PN	Practice Nurse – nurse in a GP surgery.
PRN	'Pro re nata' – medication instruction to give 'as and when required'.

PUFO	Pissed up fell over – not official terminology. You didn't hear it from me.
RN / RGN	Registered Nurse / Registered General Nurse. My title.
SDTI	Suspected Deep Tissue Injury – pressure damage that appears as a dark bruise but you don't know the extent of the damage underneath.
'Trained'	Registered nurse. Used alongside 'untrained' to differentiate between registered and unregistered staff. Untrained are actually quite highly trained in their band so it's a term that shouldn't really be used.
TWOC	Trial Without Catheter – the process followed when removing a long-term urinary catheter.
UTI	Urinary Tract Infection – 'water infection'.
VTD	Visit, Treat, Discharge – one off simple patients who don't need ongoing care. For example, stitch removal.